GETTING STARTED WITH THE MULTIPLE SCLEROSIS DIET

Everything You Need to Know About MS Disease Treatments, Diet Plans to Prevent Inflammation, and Support Immune Health

Chris Preston, RDN

ACKNOWLEDGEMENTS

I would like to express my deepest gratitude to everyone who supported me throughout the journey of creating this book. To my family and friends, your unwavering encouragement and patience have been invaluable.

A special thanks to my team, whose expertise and guidance were crucial in developing the dietary plans and recipes shared in this book. Your insights have been a cornerstone of this work.

I am also deeply grateful to my editor, Michael Jones, for your meticulous attention to detail and for helping shape this book into a comprehensive and accessible guide.

To the support groups and communities who shared their experiences and provided feedback, your contributions have enriched this book and made it more relatable for those living with fructose intolerance.

Lastly, to my readers, thank you for embarking on this journey with me. I hope this book provides you with the knowledge and tools to navigate your dietary needs and improve your quality of life.

COPYRIGHT

This book is intended to provide general information about diet and nutrition. It is not intended as a substitute for professional medical advice, diagnosis, or treatment. Always seek the advice of your physician or other qualified health provider with any questions you may have regarding a medical condition.

TABLE OF CONTENTS

PART I

INTRODUCTION TO MULTIPLE SCLEROSIS DIET

Multiple sclerosis (MS) is a long-lasting chronic disease that affects the central nervous system, including the brain, spinal cord, and optic nerves. Symptoms can range from muscle weakness to vision loss. They tend to worsen during flares and improve during times of remission.

It is not possible to predict how multiple sclerosis (MS) will progress in any individual.

Some people have mild symptoms, such as blurred vision and numbness, and tingling in the limbs. In severe cases, a person may experience paralysis, vision loss, and mobility problems. However, this is not common.

It is difficult to know precisely how many people have MS. According to the National Institute for Neurological Disorders and Stroke (NINDS), 250,000–350,000Trusted Source people in the United States are living with MS.

The National Multiple Sclerosis Society estimates the number could be closer to 1 million.

New treatments are proving effective at slowing the disease.

Scientists do not know exactly what causes MS, but they believe it is an autoimmune disorder that affects the central nervous system (CNS).

When a person has an autoimmune disease, the immune system attacks healthy tissue, just as it might attack a virus or bacteria.

In the case of MS, the immune system attacks the myelin causing inflammation. Myelin is a protein and fatty substance that surrounds and protects nerve fibers. In MS, the immune system attacks the myelin, which becomes destroyed in many areas. This loss of myelin forms scar tissue called sclerosis. These areas are also called plaques or lesions. When the nerves are damaged in this way, they can't conduct electrical impulses normally to and from the brain.

Multiple sclerosis means "scar tissue in multiple areas." They mainly affect:

• the brain stem

- the cerebellum, which coordinates movement and controls balance

- the spinal cord

- the optic nerves

- white matter in some regions of the brain

As more lesions develop, nerve fibers can break or become damaged. As a result, the electrical impulses from the brain do not flow smoothly to the target nerve. This means that the body cannot carry out certain functions.

When MS causes repeated attacks, it's called relapsing remitting MS. When the symptoms progress over time without clear attacks, it's called primary progressive MS.

What are the types of MS?

Your MS may change and evolve. You can only have one type of MS at a time, but knowing when you transition to a progressive form of MS may be difficult to pinpoint.

Types of MS include:

Clinically isolated syndrome (CIS)

CIS is a pre-MS condition involving one episode of symptoms lasting at least 24 hours. These symptoms are due to demyelination in your CNS.

Although this episode is characteristic of MS, it's not enough to prompt a diagnosis. CIS can fully resolve, and a person can have a single episode without any future episodes.

If you have more than one lesion or positive oligoclonal bands (OCBs) in your spinal fluid at the time of a spinal tap, then you might be more likely to eventually be diagnosed with RRMS. If you have evidence of a previous lesion, you might be diagnosed with RRMS during the evaluation for CIS.

If these lesions are absent or your spinal fluid does not show OCBs, you are less likely to receive an MS diagnosis.

Relapsing-remitting MS (RRMS)

Relapsing-remitting MS (RRMS) involves clear relapses of disease activity followed by remissions. During remission periods, symptoms are mild or absent, and there's mild to moderate disease progression.

RRMS is the most common form of MS at diagnosis and accounts for about 85% of all initial MS diagnoses, according to the NMSS.

Primary progressive MS (PPMS)

If you have primary progressive MS (PPMS), neurological function becomes progressively worse from the onset of your symptoms.

However, short periods of stability can occur. The terms "active" and "not active" are sometimes used to describe disease activity with new or enhancing brain lesions.

Secondary progressive MS (SPMS)

Secondary progressive MS (SPMS) occurs when RRMS transitions into the progressive form. In addition to disability or gradual worsening of function, you may still have noticeable relapses.

Multiple Sclerosis Symptoms

Because MS affects the CNS, which controls all the actions in the body, symptoms can affect any part of the body.

The most common symptoms of MS are:

Muscle weakness: People may develop weak muscles due to lack of use or stimulation due to nerve damage.

Numbness and tingling: A pins and needles-type sensation is one of the earliest symptoms of MS and can affect the face, body, arms, and legs.

Lhermitte's sign: A person may experience a sensation like an electric shock when they move their neck, known as Lhermitte's sign.

Bladder problems: A person may have difficulty emptying their bladder or need to urinate frequently or suddenly, known as urge incontinence. Loss of bladder control is an early sign of MS.

Bowel problems: Constipation can cause fecal impaction, which can lead to bowel incontinence.

Fatigue: Fatigue can undermine a person's ability to function at work or at home, and is one of the most common symptoms of MS.

Dizziness and vertigo: These are common problems, along with balance and coordination issues.

Sexual dysfunction: Both males and females may lose interest in sex.

Spasticity and muscle spasms: This is an early sign of MS. Damage to nerve fibers in the spinal cord and brain can cause painful muscle spasms, including in the legs.

Tremor: Some people with MS may experience involuntary quivering movements.

Vision problems: Some people may experience double or blurred vision or a partial or total loss of vision. This usually affects one eye at a time. Inflammation of the optic nerve can result in pain when the eye moves. Vision problems are an early sign of MS.

Gait and mobility changes: MS can change the way people walk due to muscle weakness and problems with balance, dizziness, and fatigue.

Emotional changes and depression: Demyelination and nerve fiber damage in the brain can trigger emotional changes.

Learning and memory problems: These can make it difficult to concentrate, plan, learn, prioritize, and multitask.

Pain: Pain is a common symptom in MS. Neuropathic pain is directly due to MS, while muscle spasticity or stiffness may cause localized pain.

Less common symptoms include:

- Headaches
- Hearing loss
- Itching
- Respiratory or breathing problems
- Seizures
- Speech disorders

- Swallowing problems

There is also a higher risk of urinary tract infections, reduced activity, and loss of mobility. These can impact a person's work and social life.

In the later stages, people may experience changes in perception and thinking, as well as sensitivity to heat.

MS affects individuals differently. For some, it starts with a subtle sensation, and their symptoms do not progress for months or years. Sometimes, symptoms worsen rapidly, within weeks or months.

A few people will only have mild symptoms, and others will experience significant changes that lead to disability. However, most people will experience times when symptoms worsen and then get better.

Disease course

Most people with MS have a relapsing-remitting disease course. They experience periods of new symptoms or relapses that develop over days or weeks and usually improve partially or completely. These relapses are followed by quiet periods of disease remission that can last months or even years.

Small increases in body temperature can temporarily worsen signs and symptoms of MS. These aren't considered true disease relapses but pseudorelapses.

At least 20% to 40% of those with relapsing-remitting MS can eventually develop a steady progression of symptoms, with or without periods of remission, within 10 to 20 years from disease onset. This is known as secondary-progressive MS.

The worsening of symptoms usually includes problems with mobility and gait. The rate of disease progression varies greatly among people with secondary-progressive MS.

Some people with MS experience a gradual onset and steady progression of signs and symptoms without any relapses, known as primary-progressive MS.

Causes and Risk Factors

Causes

If you have MS, the protective layer of myelin around some of the nerve fibers of your brain, optic nerve, and spinal cord become damaged.

Experts think that this damage may result from an autoimmune process in which the immune system targets myelin. While more research is needed, an environmental trigger, such as a virus or toxin, may set off this process.

As your immune system damages the myelin, demyelination occurs. This can go into remission as new layers of myelin form, but chronic inflammation can lead to scar tissue, which can result in lasting neurological impairment.

MS is not hereditary, but having a parent or sibling with MS raises your risk slightly. Scientists have identified some genes that seem to increase susceptibility to developing MS, according to a review of studies published in 2011.

Experts do not know why some people develop MS. However, several risk factors may increase the risk.

Risk factors

These factors may increase your risk of developing multiple sclerosis:

Age. MS can occur at any age, but onset usually occurs around 20 and 40 years of age. However, younger and older people can be affected.

Sex. Women are more than 2 to 3 times as likely as men are to have relapsing-remitting MS.

Family history. If one of your parents or siblings has had MS, you are at higher risk of developing the disease.

Certain infections. A variety of viruses have been linked to MS, including Epstein-Barr, the virus that causes infectious mononucleosis.

Race. White people, particularly those of Northern European descent, are at highest risk of developing MS. People of Asian, African or Native American descent have the lowest risk. A recent study suggests that the number of Black and Hispanic young adults with multiple sclerosis may be greater than previously thought.

Climate. MS is far more common in countries with temperate climates, including Canada, the northern United States, New Zealand, southeastern Australia and Europe. Your birth month may also affect the chances of developing multiple sclerosis, since exposure to the sun when a mother is pregnant seems to decrease later development of multiple sclerosis in these children.

Vitamin D. Having low levels of vitamin D and low exposure to sunlight is associated with a greater risk of MS.

Your genes. A gene on chromosome 6p21 has been found to be associated with multiple sclerosis.

Obesity. An association with obesity and multiple sclerosis has been found in females. This is especially true for female childhood and adolescent obesity.

Certain autoimmune diseases. You have a slightly higher risk of developing MS if you have other autoimmune disorders such as thyroid disease, pernicious anemia, psoriasis, type 1 diabetes or inflammatory bowel disease.

Smoking. Smokers who experience an initial symptom that may signal MS are more likely than nonsmokers to develop a second event that confirms relapsing-remitting MS.

What are the complications of MS?

MS lesions can appear anywhere in your CNS and have wide-ranging effects. Many people with MS also have:

- Depression
- Anxiety
- Some degree of cognitive impairment
- Muscle spasticity or stiffness
- Muscle atrophy or thinning

If you have other medical conditions, MS can have a more substantial impact on your overall health.

If you have mobility issues, falling may increase your risk of bone fractures. Other conditions, such as arthritis and osteoporosis, can complicate matters. Mobility issues can lead to a lack of physical activity, which can cause other health problems. Fatigue and mobility issues may also have an effect on mental health.

Diagnosis and Treatment

Diagnosis

Not one specific test is used to diagnose MS. Diagnosis is based on symptoms and signs, imaging tests, and lab tests. A healthcare provider can make a diagnosis by following a careful process to rule out other causes and diseases.

Two things must be true to make a diagnosis of relapsing remitting MS:

1. You must have had 2 attacks at least 1 month apart. An attack is when any MS symptoms show up suddenly. Or when any MS symptoms get worse for at least 24 hours.

2. You must have more than 1 area of damage to the central nervous system myelin. Myelin is the sheath that surrounds and protects nerve fibers. This damage must have occurred at more than 1 point in time and not have been caused by any other disease.

Your healthcare provider will ask about your health history and do a neurological exam. This includes:

• Mental functions

- Emotional functions

- Language functions

- Movement and coordination

- Vision

- Balance

- Functions of the 5 senses

There are no specific tests for MS. Instead, a diagnosis of multiple sclerosis often relies on ruling out other conditions that might produce similar signs and symptoms, known as a differential diagnosis.

Your doctor is likely to start with a thorough medical history and examination.

Your doctor may then recommend:

- **Blood tests,** to help rule out other diseases with symptoms like MS. Tests to check for specific biomarkers associated with MS are currently under development and may also aid in diagnosing the disease.

- **Spinal tap (lumbar puncture),** in which a small sample of cerebrospinal fluid is removed from your spinal canal for laboratory analysis. This sample can show abnormalities in antibodies that are associated with MS. A spinal tap can also help rule out infections and other conditions with symptoms like MS. A new antibody test (for kappa free light chains) may be faster and less expensive than previous spinal fluid tests for multiple sclerosis.

- **MRI,** which can reveal areas of MS (lesions) on your brain, cervical and thoracic spinal cord. You may receive an intravenous injection of a contrast material to highlight lesions that indicate your disease is in an active phase.

• **Evoked potential tests** that record the electrical signals produced by your nervous system in response to stimuli may be done. An evoked potential test may use visual stimuli or electrical stimuli. In these tests, you watch a moving visual pattern, as short electrical impulses are applied to nerves in your legs or arms. Electrodes measure how quickly the information travels down your nerve pathways.

In most people with relapsing-remitting MS, the diagnosis is straightforward and based on a pattern of symptoms consistent with the disease and confirmed by brain imaging scans, such as an MRI.

Diagnosing MS can be more difficult in people with unusual symptoms or progressive disease. In these cases, further testing with spinal fluid analysis, evoked potentials and additional imaging may be needed.

Treatment

There is no cure for multiple sclerosis. Treatment typically focuses on speeding recovery from attacks, reducing new radiographic and clinical relapses, slowing the progression of the disease, and managing MS symptoms. Some people have such mild symptoms that no treatment is necessary.

Treatments for MS attacks

• **Corticosteroids**, such as oral prednisone and intravenous methylprednisolone, are prescribed to reduce nerve inflammation. Side effects may include insomnia, increased blood pressure, increased blood glucose levels, mood swings and fluid retention.

• **Plasma exchange (plasmapheresis).** The liquid portion of part of your blood (plasma) is removed and separated from your blood cells. The blood cells are then mixed with a protein solution (albumin) and put back into your body. Plasma exchange may be used if your symptoms are new, severe and haven't responded to steroids.

Treatments to modify progression

There are several disease modifying therapies (DMTs) for relapsing-remitting MS. Some of these DMTs can be of benefit for secondary progressive MS, and one is available for primary progressive MS.

Much of the immune response associated with MS occurs in the early stages of the disease. Aggressive treatment with these medications as early as possible can lower the relapse rate, slow the formation of new lesions, and potentially reduce risk of brain atrophy and disability accumulation.

Many of the disease-modifying therapies used to treat MS carry significant health risks. Selecting the right therapy for you will depend on careful consideration of many factors, including duration and severity of disease, effectiveness of previous MS treatments, other health issues, cost, and child-bearing status.

Treatment options for relapsing-remitting MS include injectable, oral and infusions medications.

Injectable treatments include:

• **Interferon beta medications.** These drugs used to be the most prescribed medications to treat MS. They work by interfering with diseases that attack the body and may decrease inflammation and increase nerve growth. They are injected under the skin or into muscle and can reduce the frequency and severity of relapses.

Side effects of interferons may include flu-like symptoms and injection-site reactions. You'll need blood tests to monitor your liver enzymes because liver damage is a possible side effect of interferon use. People taking interferons may develop neutralizing antibodies that can reduce drug effectiveness.

• **Glatiramer acetate (Copaxone, Glatopa).** This medication may help block your immune system's attack on myelin and must be injected beneath the skin. Side effects may include skin irritation at the injection site.

•	**Monoclonal antibodies.** Ofatumumab (Kesimpta, Arzerra) targets cells that damage the nervous system. These cells are called B cells. Ofatumumab is given by an injection under the skin and can decrease multiple sclerosis brain lesions and worsening symptoms. Possible side effects are infections, local reactions to the injection and headaches.

Oral treatments include:

• **Teriflunomide (Aubagio).** This once-daily oral medication can reduce relapse rate. Teriflunomide can cause liver damage, hair loss and other side effects. This drug is associated with birth defects when taken by both men and women. Therefore, use contraception when taking this medication and for up to two years afterward. Couples who wish to become pregnant should talk to their doctor about ways to speed elimination of the drug from the body. This drug requires blood test monitoring on a regular basis.

- **Dimethyl fumarate (Tecfidera).** This twice-daily oral medication can reduce relapses. Side effects may include flushing, diarrhea, nausea and lowered white blood cell count. This drug requires blood test monitoring on a regular basis.

- **Diroximel fumarate (Vumerity).** This twice-daily capsule is similar to dimethyl fumarate but typically causes fewer side effects. It's approved for the treatment of relapsing forms of MS.

- **Monomethyl fumarate (Bafiertam)** was approved by the FDA as a delayed release medicine that has a slow and steady action.

Because of its time release, it is hoped that side effects will be decreased. Possible side effects are flushing, liver injury, abdominal pain and infections.

- **Fingolimod (Gilenya).** This once-daily oral medication reduces relapse rate.

You'll need to have your heart rate and blood pressure monitored for six hours after the first dose because your heart rate may be slowed. Other side effects include rare serious infections, headaches, high blood pressure and blurred vision.

- **Siponimod (Mayzent).** Research shows that this once-daily oral medication can reduce relapse rates and help slow progression of MS. It's also approved for secondary-progressive MS. Possible side effects include viral infections, liver problems and low white blood cell count. Other possible side effects include changes in heart rate, headaches and vision problems. Siponimod is harmful to a developing fetus, so women who may become pregnant should use contraception when taking this medication and for 10 days after stopping the medication. Some might need to have the heart rate and blood pressure monitored for six hours after the first dose. This drug requires blood test monitoring on a regular basis.

• **Ozanimod (Zeposia).** This oral medication decreases the relapse rate of multiple sclerosis and is given once a day. Possible side effects are an elevated blood pressure, infections and liver inflammation.

• **Ponesimod (Ponvory).** This oral medication is taken once a day with a gradually increasing dosing schedule. This medicine has a low relapse rate and has demonstrated fewer brain lesions than some other medications used to treat multiple sclerosis. The possible side effects are respiratory tract infections, high blood pressure, liver irritation and electrical problems in the heart that affect heart rate and rhythm.

• **Cladribine (Mavenclad).** This medication is generally prescribed as a second line treatment for those with relapsing-remitting MS. It was also approved for secondary-progressive MS. It is given in two treatment courses, spread over a two-week period, over the course of two years. Side effects include upper respiratory infections, headaches, tumors, serious infections and reduced levels of white blood cells. People who have active chronic infections or cancer should not take this drug, nor should women who are pregnant or breastfeeding. Men and women should use contraception when taking this medication and for the following six months. You may need monitoring with blood tests while taking cladribine.

Infusion treatments include:

• **Natalizumab (Tysabri).** This is a monoclonal antibody that has been shown to decrease relapse rates and slow down the risk of disability.

This medication is designed to block the movement of potentially damaging immune cells from your bloodstream to your brain and spinal cord. It may be considered a first line treatment for some people with severe MS or as a second line treatment in others.

This medication increases the risk of a potentially serious viral infection of the brain called progressive multifocal leukoencephalopathy (PML) in people who are positive for antibodies to the causative agent of PML JC virus. People who don't have the antibodies have extremely low risk of PML.

• **Ocrelizumab (Ocrevus).** This treatment reduces the relapse rate and the risk of disabling progression in relapsing-remitting multiple sclerosis. It also slows the progression of the primary-progressive form of multiple sclerosis.

This humanized monoclonal antibody medication is the only DMT approved by the FDA to treat both the relapse-remitting and primary-progressive forms of MS. Clinical trials showed that it reduced relapse rate in relapsing disease and slowed worsening of disability in both forms of the disease.

Ocrelizumab is given via an intravenous infusion by a medical professional. Infusion-related side effects may include irritation at the injection site, low blood pressure, a fever and nausea, among others. Some people may not be able to take ocrelizumab, including those with a hepatitis B infection. Ocrelizumab may also increase the risk of infections and some types of cancer, particularly breast cancer.

• **Alemtuzumab (Campath, Lemtrada).** This treatment is a monoclonal antibody that decreases annual relapse rates and demonstrates MRI benefits.

This drug helps reduce relapses of MS by targeting a protein on the surface of immune cells and depleting white blood cells. This effect can limit potential nerve damage caused by the white blood cells. But it also increases the risk of infections and autoimmune disorders, including a high risk of thyroid autoimmune diseases and rare immune mediated kidney disease.

Treatment with alemtuzumab involves five consecutive days of drug infusions followed by another three days of infusions a year later. Infusion reactions are common with alemtuzumab.

The drug is only available from registered providers, and people treated with the drug must be registered in a special drug safety monitoring program. Alemtuzumab is usually recommended for those with aggressive MS or as second line treatment for patients who failed another MS medication.

Treatments for MS signs and symptoms

Physical therapy for multiple sclerosis

Physical therapy can build muscle strength and ease some of the symptoms of MS.

- **Therapy.** A physical or occupational therapist can teach you stretching and strengthening exercises and show you how to use devices to make it easier to perform daily tasks.

Physical therapy along with the use of a mobility aid, when necessary, can also help manage leg weakness and other gait problems often associated with MS.

- **Muscle relaxants.** You may experience painful or uncontrollable muscle stiffness or spasms, particularly in your legs. Muscle relaxants such as baclofen (Lioresal, Gablofen), tizanidine (Zanaflex) and cyclobenzaprine may help. Onabotulinumtoxin A treatment is another option in those with spasticity.

- **Medications to reduce fatigue.** Amantadine (Gocovri, Osmolex), modafinil (Provigil) and methylphenidate (Ritalin) have been used to reduce MS-related fatigue. However, a recent study did not find amantadine, modafinil or methylphenidate to be superior to a placebo in improving MS-related fatigue and caused more frequent adverse events. Some drugs used to treat depression, including selective serotonin reuptake inhibitors, may be recommended.

- **Medication to increase walking speed.** Dalfampridine (Ampyra) may help to slightly increase walking speed in some people. Possible side effects are urinary tract infections, vertigo, insomnia and headaches. People with a history of seizures or kidney dysfunction should not take this medication.

• **Other medications.** Medications also may be prescribed for depression, pain, sexual dysfunction, insomnia, and bladder or bowel control problems that are associated with MS.

Multiple Sclerosis Prevention

MS cannot be entirely prevented. It's caused by a variety of known and unknown factors, many of which are out of your control. But there are ways to reduce your risk. Lifestyle habits such as getting adequate vitamin D, maintaining a healthy weight, living in a sunny climate, spending time outside, reducing stress, and not smoking may help prevent MS.

Recent developments or emerging therapies

Bruton's tyrosine kinase (BTK) inhibitor is an emerging therapy being studied in relapsing-remitting multiple sclerosis and secondary-progressive multiple sclerosis. It works by mostly modulating B cells, which are immune cells in the central nervous system.

Stem cell transplantation destroys the immune system of someone with multiple sclerosis and then replaces it with transplanted healthy stem cells. Researchers are still investigating whether this therapy can decrease inflammation in people with multiple sclerosis and help to "reset" the immune system. Possible side effects are fever and infections.

Researchers are learning more about how existing disease modifying therapies work to lessen relapses and reduce multiple sclerosis-related lesions in the brain. Further studies will determine whether treatment can delay disability caused by the disease.

For primary-progressive MS, ocrelizumab (Ocrevus) is the only FDA-approved disease-modifying therapy (DMT). Those who receive this treatment are slightly less likely to progress than those who are untreated.

For secondary progressive MS, some might consider the use of FDA-approved disease modifying therapies such as ozanimod, siponimod and cladribine, which can potentially slow down disabilities.

PART II

MULTIPLE SCLEROSIS AND DIET

Diet has a wide range of effects on an individual's health — it impacts a person's weight, and can alter the risk of heart disease, bone problems, and other health issues. Diet also can change the activity of the microbes that live in the digestive tract, and some substances consumed in the diet and/or made by these microbes can alter inflammation and brain activity.

There is no evidence that any one dietary strategy is best for people with MS. Generally, its recommended patients eat a varied and well-balanced diet along the lines of what is typically recommended in the general population — lots of plant-derived foods like fruits, vegetables, and whole grains, and fewer foods that are processed or high in refined sugars and fats.

People with MS are advised to work with their healthcare team to come up with a dietary plan that makes sense for them, and that's realistic given factors including personal preferences, accessibility, affordability, and cultural traditions.

While diet cannot replace treatment with MS disease-modifying therapies, studies suggest eating a balanced diet that provides for all nutritional needs may help patients better manage and control MS. Specifically, a good diet can help in:

• reducing the likelihood of flare-ups;

• lessening the chances of disability progression; and

• Improving both physical and mental health-related quality of life.

Diet also can help to ease some symptoms of the disease. For example, being obese or overweight is linked with worse severity of some MS symptoms, such as fatigue and pain. Changes to diet that help patients lose weight may ease these types of symptoms.

Dietary modifications also may be helpful for managing other specific symptoms of MS.

• Bladder problems: Drinking enough fluids to stay hydrated and avoiding spicy foods, alcohol, caffeine, and fruit juices can help with issues like frequent urination and urinary tract infections.

• Bowel problems: Eating enough fiber and drinking enough fluids can help ease constipation.

• MS fatigue: Problems related to fatigue may be worse if a person's diet isn't providing enough energy for the body to function effectively; changes in eating habits may increase vitality.

• Emotional challenges: a varied and balanced diet that avoids alcohol and caffeine may help to ease depression.

Key Nutrients for Managing MS Symptoms

Broadly speaking, it's recommended the diet for individuals with MS should be varied and well-balanced to provide all the nutrients the body needs to function. Components of a healthy diet generally include:

• Carbohydrates (sugars and starches), which are used for energy in the body;

• Proteins, used for growth and to repair damaged tissue;

• Fats, which serve as an energy source and are important for absorbing other nutrients;

• Vitamins and minerals, a broad group of essential nutrients needed for a range of bodily functions; and

• Fiber, an indigestible plant matter that helps food pass through the intestines.

Some specific nutrients of particular relevance to MS include:

• **Vitamin B12:** This vitamin is used to make myelin, the fatty wrapping around nerve fibers that becomes damaged in MS. While a deficiency in this vitamin may result in MS-like symptoms, there is no evidence that B12 supplements benefit MS patients with normal levels of the vitamin.

• **Vitamin D:** Affecting a number of biological functions, this vitamin is known to impact immune activity. Low vitamin D levels have been linked with an increased risk of MS and more severe disease activity.

• **Calcium**: This mineral is needed to maintain healthy bones. Calcium supplements may be given to MS patients at risk of bone problems — for example, individuals who have limited mobility or are taking steroid medications.

• **Essential fatty acids (EFAs):** EFAs are a class of polyunsaturated fats that cannot be synthesized in the body and must be acquired through diet. They are needed to repair damaged nerve cells and to produce certain signaling molecules that control inflammation. There are two main types of EFAs — omega 3 and omega 6 fatty acids.

• **Antioxidants**: Oxidative stress is a type of cell damage that contributes to inflammation in MS. Antioxidants, as their name suggests, are molecules that can lessen oxidative stress, thereby helping to reduce inflammation and neuronal damage. Common antioxidants include vitamins A, C, and E, as well as compounds such as flavonoids and beta-carotenes.

The Role of Fiber in MS Management

1. **Gut Microbiota Modulation**: Fibre is essential for promoting a healthy gut microbiota. A diverse and balanced gut microbiome has been

increasingly recognized as important in MS management. Studies suggest that certain gut bacteria may influence immune responses and inflammation, which are key factors in MS progression. Fibre acts as a prebiotic, feeding beneficial gut bacteria and promoting their growth, which can potentially influence the immune system in a favorable way.

2. Anti-inflammatory Effects: Fibre-rich diets, particularly those high in fruits, vegetables, and whole grains, are associated with lower levels of inflammation in the body. In MS, chronic inflammation in the central nervous system (CNS) contributes to the progression of the disease. By reducing systemic inflammation, fibre may help mitigate some of the inflammatory processes associated with MS.

3. Regulation of Blood Sugar and Insulin Levels:
Diets high in refined carbohydrates can lead to spikes in blood sugar levels and insulin resistance. High-fibre foods, such as whole grains and legumes, can help regulate blood sugar levels and improve insulin sensitivity. This is important because insulin resistance and high blood sugar levels may exacerbate inflammation and oxidative stress, which are detrimental in MS.

4. Heart Health and Weight Management:
Individuals with MS have an increased risk of cardiovascular disease. Fibre-rich diets can help lower cholesterol levels, improve heart health, and aid in weight management. Maintaining a healthy weight and cardiovascular system can have indirect benefits for individuals with MS by reducing secondary complications and improving overall well-being.

5. Symptom Management: Some MS symptoms, such as constipation, can be managed with dietary fibre. Adequate fibre intake promotes regular bowel movements and prevents constipation, which is a common issue for individuals with MS, often exacerbated by medications or reduced physical activity.

PART

FOODS TO INCLUDE AND AVOID IN AN MS DIET

Most fruits and vegetables are a good source of carbohydrates, vitamins, minerals, antioxidants, and fiber. A higher intake of fruits and veggies has been linked with less disease activity and disability among MS patients.

Whole grains

Whole grains are a good source of complex carbohydrates and fiber. Research has linked more whole grain intake with less severe MS-related disability.

Lean protein

Skinless chicken, fish, and plant-based proteins such as beans, peas, lentils, and soy products, are different kinds of lean proteins. All are considered good foods to eat to get protein without consuming a lot of saturated fats, which have been linked to more severe disease among MS patients.

Unsaturated fats

Unsaturated fats, particularly polyunsaturated fatty acids or PUFAs — which include EFAs — have been shown to have anti-inflammatory and nerve-protecting properties in animal studies. Of note, studies of PUFA intake in MS patients have shown inconsistent results. Foods rich in PUFAs and EFAs include oily fish like salmon and mackerel, and some nuts and seeds like walnuts, soybeans, and flax seed.

Another kind of unsaturated fat, monounsaturated fatty acids or MUFAs, are found in food like avocados, peanut butter, and vegetable oils. These are less well-studied in MS but have been tied to a reduced risk of heart disease in the general population.

Water

Staying hydrated is critical for maintaining health, and regularly drinking enough water can help to ease constipation and avoid bladder infections.

Foods to Avoid or Limit

Saturated fats

Considered unhealthy fats, saturated fats have been linked to an increased risk of heart disease; they also have pro-inflammatory effects. In animal models of MS, eating a diet high in saturated fat leads to more inflammation, and higher saturated fat intake has been linked with increased relapse risk and more disability among MS patients. Saturated fats are mainly found in animal-based foods such as whole milk, high-fat cheese, pastries, cured meats, and fatty cuts of meat. Some plant-based foods such as coconut oil, palm oils, and cocoa butter also are high in saturated fat.

Trans fats

Trans fats are strongly associated with an increased risk of heart disease, so most experts recommend limiting the amount included in the diet. Fried foods, commercial baked goods, frozen pizza, margarine and other shortening foods, and processed foods commonly have a high trans fat content.

Refined sugar

The effects of a high-sugar diet — containing a lot of sweetened beverages and cereals, cookies, and cakes — have not been confirmed in studies of people with MS. But a high sugar intake can promote inflammation and lead to more aggressive disease in MS mouse models. A small study found that MS patients who drink more sugar-sweetened beverages like soda tend to have more severe disease. High sugar intake also is linked with a higher risk of other conditions, like diabetes and heart disease, which may exacerbate the symptoms of MS.

Alcohol

Evidence suggests the overall severity of MS is not affected by alcohol intake. However, especially in large quantities, alcohol's effects on the body can cause worsening of numerous MS symptoms, including coordination difficulties, bladder problems, and depression. Alcohol also may interact with medications. Consequently, it's generally recommended that people with MS should practice moderation in their alcohol intake, and should discuss how much alcohol it is safe to consume with their healthcare teams.

More research needed

Dairy

It remains unclear whether consuming dairy products affects the course of MS. Some studies have found MS patients who consume more dairy tend to have more severe disease, but other studies have reported the exact opposite trend, with more dairy consumption linked to less severe MS. Full-fat dairy products are often high in saturated fats, but dairy also can be a good source of protein, calcium, and vitamin D. Some experts recommend MS patients stick with low-fat dairy options or dairy alternatives, which include products made from nuts, soy, and oats.

There is experimental evidence that an immune system attack against a protein found in cow's milk can lead to MS-like autoimmunity in the nervous system, but the clinical relevance of these findings for people with MS is unclear.

Salt

Some research has suggested a link between higher salt (sodium) intake and more severe MS, but other studies have shown no connection between salt consumption and MS severity. A high-salt diet can increase the risk of other health problems like high blood pressure, so it's generally recommended that salt in the diet be moderated.

Gluten

A few studies have explored whether gluten intake may influence MS, but there is not enough evidence to make any conclusions one way or another. Available evidence suggests the rate of gluten intolerance, known as celiac disease, is no higher among MS patients than in the general population.

Vitamin D

Vitamin D is mostly produced in the skin upon sun exposure but also can be obtained in the diet through food or supplements. This vitamin is important for maintaining bone health, and also can modulate the activity of the immune and nervous systems.

A deficiency in vitamin D has been linked with an increased risk of MS, and patients commonly have lower-than-normal levels of this vitamin. In MS patients with low vitamin D levels, supplements or other interventions that aim to normalize vitamin D levels are generally recommended.

Some studies have tested whether additional vitamin D supplementation may provide benefits to MS patients. So far, however, the data have not shown any clear benefit of vitamin D supplements beyond maintaining normal levels. Clinical trials in MS patients also suggest that high doses of vitamin D supplementation bring no added benefit over lower doses.

Special diets for Multiple Sclerosis

There is no single diet universally recommended for people with MS. Still, several dietary strategies have been developed for multiple sclerosis, which generally aim to provide for the body's nutritional needs while avoiding foods that could worsen inflammation.

Some of these diets have been explored in clinical trials, but studies are generally small, lack comparison groups, and often have high dropout rates. These factors can make it hard to determine how meaningful the results are.

It's also important to keep in mind that researching the impacts of diet among people is necessarily complicated, given the other factors at play — from genetics to lifestyle, and even whether or not someone chooses to participate in clinical research — that may affect the results.

Best Bet diet

The Best Bet diet is based on the idea that molecules in certain foods may leak out of the intestines and worsen the inflammatory attack that drives MS. It is a strict exclusion diet that recommends cutting out all dairy, grains, legumes, sugar-rich foods, and any foods that may cause an allergic reaction, such as eggs and yeast. It also recommends reducing the intake of saturated and polyunsaturated fats, salt, and alcohol.

Developed by Ashton Embry, a geologist whose son has MS, the diet consists mainly of fish and lean meats, lots of fruits and vegetables, and olive oil. It also recommends a number of nutritional supplements, such as vitamin D, calcium, magnesium, and omega 3 fatty acids.

While some people with MS report feeling better on this diet, there is no research showing benefit for MS patients. Because the diet cuts out many food groups, it's important that any MS patients following it should take precautions to ensure they get all needed nutrients.

Ketogenic diet

A ketogenic or "keto" diet is one that is low in carbohydrates and high in fats, leading the body to use fats as its main energy source — a process called ketosis. The diet was originally developed to help manage certain seizure-causing disorders.

A few small studies have indicated that following a keto diet may help to ease fatigue and depression, and improve quality of life in people with MS. However, the diet also may have negative effects, like vitamin deficiencies or digestive upset. In rare cases, it can cause serious problems with the pancreas and liver.

McDougall diet

The McDougall diet is a low-fat, plant-based diet rich in complex carbohydrates, whole grains, fruits, and vegetables. It completely cuts out meat, dairy, oils, and all other foods that come from animals, and only allows small amounts of sugar and salt.

In studies, the McDougall diet has not shown any effect on measures of MS progression, such as relapse rates or inflammatory activity on MRI scans. But some research suggests the diet may help ease fatigue in MS patients.

Mediterranean diet

As its name suggests, the Mediterranean diet is based on the foods that are commonly eaten in cultures surrounding the Mediterranean Sea. The diet includes plenty of fruits and veggies, whole grains, and olive oil, and recommends a moderate amount of low-fat dairy products, fish, poultry, and red wine. Only limited amounts of red meat, sweets, and animal fats are included in this diet.

There is not much research specifically evaluating the Mediterranean diet in MS, though the plan is generally considered well-balanced and nutritionally complete. Some small studies suggest it could help ease fatigue, as well as reduce the impact of MS symptoms and delay disability progression.

Overcoming MS diet

The overcoming MS (OMS) diet is a plant-based diet that also includes fish and seafood, but cuts out all processed foods, eggs, meat, dairy, and saturated fats. The diet usually includes daily supplements of flaxseed oil or fish oil. Additional supplements or dietary modifications may be needed to ensure patients get enough nutrients, like protein, iron, and calcium.

The diet was developed by George Jelinek, MD, an Australian doctor who was diagnosed with MS in the late 1990s, as part of a lifestyle program that includes diet, exercise, and meditation, alongside medical treatment.

A few small studies have reported that this diet or lifestyle intervention is associated with increased mental and physical quality of life, and a columnist with Multiple Sclerosis News Today also reported feeling better just a few weeks into the diet. But the studies usually lack a comparison group so it's difficult to draw firm conclusions.

Paleo diet and the Wahls protocol

The paleolithic or Paleo diet involves eating foods that are thought to be similar to what ancient humans ate before the advent of farming and agriculture. The diet mainly includes meats, fish, nuts, vegetables, and fruits, while it excludes processed foods, grains and beans, potatoes, cereals, dairy, and eggs.

The Wahls protocol is a lifestyle intervention that combines a Paleo-inspired diet with vitamins, meditation, and exercise. The protocol is named for Terry Wahls, MD, an American doctor with MS who promoted it.

There is some evidence that a Paleo or Wahls diet can help to ease fatigue and improve quality of life in people with MS. However, because the diet cuts out many large groups of food, it may increase the risk of nutritional insufficiencies, so it's important that patients work with their care team to ensure that their nutritional needs are being adequately met.

Swank diet

The Swank diet mainly advocates strictly limiting fat intake, emphasizing low-fat dairy products, whole-grain starches, fruits, and veggies, and cutting out red meats and oily fish. Proposed in 1948 by neurologist Roy Swank, MD, PhD, the diet also recommends cod liver oil and vitamin supplements to ensure patients meet all their nutritional requirements.

A study conducted by Swank more than 30 years ago suggested that people who followed the diet had lower risk of relapse, disability, and mortality than those who didn't. But the study did not include a control group or a scoring system for MS disability, so the meaningfulness of these results is debatable. More recently, a small 2021 clinical trial suggested the Swank diet may ease fatigue and improve physical quality of life in MS patients.

PART

DELICIOUSLY SIMPLE RECIPES YOU MUST TRY!

BREAKFAST RECIPES FOR MULTIPLE SCLEROSIS

Copycat Starbucks Spinach & Mushroom Egg Bites

Ingredients

- 1 tablespoon extra-virgin olive oil

- 1 ½ cups sliced cremini mushrooms

- 3 cups packed baby spinach

- ½ teaspoon kosher salt, divided

- 8 large eggs

- ¾ cup nonfat cottage cheese

- ½ teaspoon cracked black pepper

- ¼ cup shredded Swiss cheese

Directions

1. Preheat oven to 350°F. Lightly coat a 12-cup silicone muffin pan with cooking spray; place on top of a large rimmed baking sheet.

2. Heat oil in a large skillet over medium heat. Add mushrooms; cook, stirring occasionally, until browned, 6 to 8 minutes. Add spinach; cook, stirring often, until wilted, about 1 minute. Stir in 1/4 teaspoon salt. Remove from heat and let cool for 5 minutes.

3. Transfer the spinach mixture to a food processor; pulse until the vegetables are very finely chopped. Divide the mixture evenly among the prepared muffin cups, about 1 tablespoon each. Wipe the food processor clean.

4. Add eggs, cottage cheese, pepper and the remaining 1/4 teaspoon salt to the food processor. Process on medium speed until smooth, about 20 seconds. Add Swiss cheese and pulse a few more times to incorporate. Divide the mixture among the muffin cups, a scant 1/4 cup each.

5. Bring 2 cups water to a boil. Transfer the baking sheet to the oven and carefully pour the boiling water onto the baking sheet around the muffin pan. Bake until the eggs are set, about 25 minutes. Let cool for 5 minutes before removing from the pan.

Sheet-Pan Banana Pancakes

Ingredients

• 2 overripe bananas

• 2 large eggs

• 1 cup water

• 1 teaspoon cinnamon

• 2 cups high-protein buttermilk pancake and waffle mix

Directions

1. Preheat oven to 425°F. Coat a 13-by 9-inch baking pan or baking sheet with cooking spray, then line with parchment paper and coat again.

2. Mash bananas in a large bowl. Whisk in eggs, water and cinnamon. Use a wooden spoon to fold in pancake mix; stir until just combined.

3. Spread the batter in an even layer in the prepared pan. Bake until a toothpick inserted in the center comes out clean, 12 to 14 minutes. Let cool in the pan for 3 minutes, then cut into 12 squares.

Make-Ahead Freezer Breakfast Burritos with Eggs, Cheese & Spinach

Ingredients

- 12 large eggs

- ¼ teaspoon salt

- ¼ teaspoon ground pepper

- 2 teaspoons extra-virgin olive oil

- 1 tablespoon finely chopped seeded serrano pepper

- ½ teaspoon paprika

- 2 cups baby spinach

- 6 (8 inch) whole-wheat tortillas

- ½ cup shredded pepper Jack cheese

Directions

1. Whisk eggs, salt and pepper in a large bowl.

2. Heat oil in a large nonstick pan over medium-low heat. Add serrano and paprika; cook, stirring frequently, until fragrant, 1 to 2 minutes. Add spinach; cook, stirring occasionally, until wilted, 1 to 2 minutes. Pour in the eggs and cook, stirring

occasionally, until the eggs are mostly set, about 5 minutes,

3. To assemble burritos, place each tortilla on a sheet of foil. Add ½ cup scrambled eggs to the bottom half of the tortilla, then divide cheese evenly (about 1 tablespoon + 1 teaspoon per burrito). Roll snugly, tucking in the ends as you go. Wrap tightly in the foil and freeze for up to 3 months.

4. To reheat, unwrap a burrito and transfer to a microwave-safe plate. Cover with a paper towel and microwave on Medium (or 50% or Defrost) for 1 to 2 minutes. Microwave on High until heated through, about 2 minutes. (Alternatively, bake foil-wrapped burritos at 375°F until heated through, about 25 minutes.)

Classic Breakfast Banana Split

Ingredients

- ¼ cup almond butter

- 1 tablespoon cacao powder

- 3 tablespoons water

- 2 tablespoons pure maple syrup, divided

- ¼ cup heavy cream

- 4 ripe bananas, peeled and halved lengthwise

- ⅔ cup low-fat vanilla strained yogurt

- ⅔ cup low-fat strawberry strained yogurt

- ⅔ cup whole-milk chocolate strained yogurt (see **Tip**)

- ½ cup pitted cherries

- 4 tablespoons granola

Directions

1. Whisk almond butter, cacao powder, water and 1 tablespoon maple syrup in a small bowl until smooth.

2. Whisk cream and the remaining 1 tablespoon maple syrup in a small bowl until soft peaks form.

3. Arrange 2 banana halves on each of 4 plates. Use an ice-cream scoop to divide vanilla, strawberry and chocolate yogurts among the bananas. Drizzle the almond sauce over the yogurt. Divide cherries and granola among the banana splits. Top with the whipped cream.

Tip

To make your own chocolate yogurt, stir 1 Tbsp. cocoa powder into 2/3 cup vanilla strained yogurt.

Baked Oatmeal with Banana, Raisins & Walnuts

Ingredients

- 2 cups rolled oats

- ⅓ cup walnuts, chopped

- 1 ½ teaspoons ground cinnamon

- 1 teaspoon baking powder

- ½ teaspoon salt

- ¼ teaspoon ground allspice

- 2 cups reduced-fat milk

- ¾ cup low-fat plain yogurt

- 2 tablespoons canola oil

- ¼ cup packed light brown sugar

- 1 teaspoon vanilla extract

- 1 large banana, halved lengthwise and sliced

- ⅓ cup raisins

Directions

1. Preheat oven to 375°F. Coat an 8-inch-square baking dish with cooking spray.

2. Mix oats, walnuts, cinnamon, baking powder, salt and allspice in a large bowl. Combine milk, yogurt, oil, brown sugar and vanilla in a medium bowl. Add the milk mixture to the dry Ingredients; stir until completely incorporated.

Stir in bananas and raisins. Pour the mixture into the prepared baking dish.

3. Bake until golden on top and firm to the touch, 45 to 50 minutes.

Avocado Toast with Egg, Spinach & Salsa

Ingredients

- ½ small avocado, mashed

- 1 slice whole-grain bread, toasted

- Pinch of ground pepper

- 1 teaspoon extra-virgin olive oil, divided

- 1 clove garlic, minced

- 2 cups baby spinach

- 1 large egg

- 1 tablespoon salsa

Directions

1. Spread avocado on toast; season with pepper.

2. Heat 1/2 teaspoon oil in a small nonstick skillet over medium heat. Add garlic and spinach and cook, stirring, until the spinach is wilted, 30 to 60 seconds. Top the avocado toast with the spinach.

3. Heat the remaining 1/2 teaspoon oil in the pan. Crack egg into the pan. Reduce heat to medium-low and cook 5 to 7 minutes for a soft-set yolk. Top the toast with the egg and salsa.

Vegan Chickpea Omelet

Ingredients

- ⅓ cup chickpea flour

- ⅓ cup water

- 1 ½ teaspoons nutritional yeast

- ¼ teaspoon baking powder

- ⅛ teaspoon garlic powder

- ⅛ teaspoon onion powder

- ⅛ teaspoon ground turmeric

- ⅛ teaspoon kala namak (see **Tip**)

- 1 tablespoon extra-virgin olive oil, divided

- ¾ cup mixed cooked vegetables (such as bell peppers, onions and/or mushrooms), vegan cheese, chopped fresh herbs and/or vegan meat substitutes, for toppings (optional)

Directions

1. Whisk chickpea flour, water, nutritional yeast, baking powder, garlic powder, onion powder, turmeric, kala namak and 1 1/2 teaspoons of oil in a small bowl until smooth. Let stand for 5 minutes.

2. Heat the remaining 1 1/2 teaspoons oil in a medium nonstick skillet over medium heat; swirl to coat the pan. Pour in the chickpea mixture. Cook, undisturbed, until the top is covered in bubbles and looks dry, about 4 minutes. Remove from heat.

3. If desired, spread toppings of choice over half of the omelet. Using a spatula, fold the omelet over the filling (or simply fold the omelet in half, if not using toppings). Cover the pan; let stand to

steam for 5 minutes. Slide the omelet onto a plate to serve.

Tip

Kala namak, or black salt, helps add an eggy flavor to this dish while still keeping it vegan. You can buy kala namak from retailers like The Spice Lab, or substitute regular salt.

Banana-Bran Muffins

Ingredients

• 2 large eggs

• ⅔ cup packed light brown sugar

• 1 cup mashed ripe bananas, (2 medium)

• 1 cup buttermilk, (see Ingredient notes)

- 1 cup unprocessed wheat bran, (see Ingredient notes)

- ¼ cup canola oil

- 1 teaspoon vanilla extract

- 1 cup whole-wheat flour

- ¾ cup all-purpose flour

- 1 ½ teaspoons baking powder

- ½ teaspoon baking soda

- ½ teaspoon ground cinnamon

- ¼ teaspoon salt

- ½ cup chocolate chips (optional)

- ⅓ cup chopped walnuts (optional)

Directions

1. Preheat oven to 400°F. Coat 12 muffin cups with cooking spray.

2. Whisk eggs and brown sugar in a medium bowl until smooth. Whisk in bananas, buttermilk, wheat bran, oil and vanilla.

3. Whisk whole-wheat flour, all-purpose flour, baking powder, baking soda, cinnamon and salt in a large bowl. Make a well in the dry Ingredients; add the wet Ingredients and stir with a rubber spatula until just combined. Stir in chocolate chips, if using. Scoop the batter into the prepared muffin cups (they'll be quite full). Sprinkle with walnuts, if using.

4. Bake the muffins until the tops are golden brown and spring back when touched lightly, 15 to 25 minutes. Let cool in the pan for 5 minutes.

Loosen the edges and turn the muffins out onto a wire rack to cool slightly before serving.

Avocado & Smoked Salmon Omelet

Ingredients

- 2 large eggs

- 1 teaspoon low-fat milk

- Pinch of salt

- 1 teaspoon extra-virgin olive oil plus 1/2 teaspoon, divided

- ¼ avocado, sliced

- 1 ounce smoked salmon

- 1 tablespoon chopped fresh basil

Directions

1. Beat eggs with milk and salt in a small bowl. Heat 1 teaspoon oil in a small nonstick skillet over medium heat. Add the egg mixture and cook until the bottom is set and the center is still a bit runny, 1 to 2 minutes. Flip the omelet over and cook until set, about 30 seconds more. Transfer to a plate. Top with avocado, salmon and basil. Drizzle with the remaining 1/2 teaspoon oil.

Peanut Butter Energy Balls

Ingredients

- 2 cups rolled oats

- 1 cup natural peanut butter or other nut butter

- ½ cup honey

- ¼ cup mini chocolate chips

- ¼ cup unsweetened shredded coconut

Directions

1. Combine oats, peanut butter (or other nut butter), honey, chocolate chips and coconut in a medium bowl; stir well. Using a 1-tablespoon measure, roll the mixture into balls.

Spinach & Feta Scrambled Egg Pitas

Ingredients

- 1 tablespoon extra-virgin olive oil

- 1 (10 ounce) block frozen chopped spinach, thawed, drained and squeezed dry

- Pinch salt

- 8 large eggs, beaten

- ¼ cup finely crumbled feta cheese

- Freshly ground pepper to taste

- 8 teaspoons sun-dried tomato tapenade or sun-dried tomato pesto

- 4 whole-wheat pitas (5-inch), cut in half, warmed if desired

Directions

1. Heat oil in a large nonstick skillet over medium heat. Add spinach and salt and cook until steaming hot, stirring occasionally. Add eggs and cook, stirring the eggs as they set, until they form soft curds and are just moist, 4 to 5 minutes. Add feta and pepper and cook until set.

2. Spread tapenade (or pesto) inside pita pockets, 2 teaspoons per pita. Divide the egg mixture among the pitas.

Breakfast Lemon, Raspberry & Cream Cheese Oatmeal Cakes

Ingredients

- ¼ cup reduced-fat cream cheese

- 1 tablespoon raspberry jam

- 1 teaspoon finely grated lemon zest

- 1 teaspoon fresh lemon juice

- 3 cups old-fashioned rolled oats

- 1 ¼ cups low-fat milk

- 1 cup fresh or frozen raspberries, divided

- ⅓ cup packed brown sugar

- ¼ cup unsweetened applesauce

- 2 large eggs, lightly beaten

- 1 teaspoon baking powder

- 1 teaspoon vanilla extract

- ½ teaspoon salt

Directions

1. Preheat oven to 375°F. Coat a 12-cup muffin tin with cooking spray.

2. Whisk cream cheese, jam and lemon juice together in a small bowl.

3. Combine oats, milk, 1/2 cup raspberries, brown sugar, applesauce, eggs, baking powder, vanilla, lemon zest and salt in a large bowl,

breaking up the raspberries to distribute them throughout the batter. Fill each of the prepared muffin cups with 2 to 3 tablespoons batter, then top with a dollop of the raspberry cream cheese and some of the remaining 1/2 cup raspberries. Cover with the remaining batter. Bake until a toothpick inserted in the center comes out clean, 25 to 30 minutes. Run a knife around the edges of the muffin cups to release the oatmeal cakes. Cool in the pan for 10 minutes, then turn out onto a wire rack. Serve warm or at room temperature.

Avocado Toast

Ingredients

- ½ small avocado

- ½ teaspoon lemon juice

- ⅛ teaspoon kosher salt

- ⅛ teaspoon freshly ground black pepper

- 1 slice whole-grain bread, toasted

- ½ teaspoon extra-virgin olive oil

- Flaky sea salt, such as Maldon, or crushed red pepper for garnish (optional)

Directions

1. Combine ½ avocado, ½ teaspoon lemon juice, ⅛ teaspoon salt and pepper to taste in a small bowl. Gently mash with the back of a fork.

2. Top 1 slice toasted bread with mashed avocado mixture. Drizzle with ½ teaspoon olive oil and sprinkle with Maldon sea salt and/or crushed red pepper, if desired.

Oatmeal Waffles

Ingredients

- 1 cup old-fashioned rolled oats

- 1 ½ cups all-purpose flour

- 1 teaspoon baking powder

- 1 teaspoon ground cinnamon

- ½ teaspoon salt

- 2 cups oat milk or other nondairy milk

- 2 large eggs, lightly beaten

- 6 tablespoons unsalted butter, melted

- 3 tablespoons light brown sugar

- 1 teaspoon vanilla extract

- 2 cups mixed fresh blueberries and blackberries

- Maple syrup or vanilla yogurt (optional)

Directions

1. Preheat waffle iron to medium-high. Process oats in a blender to a fine powder, about 20 seconds. Transfer to a medium bowl. Add flour, baking powder, cinnamon and salt; whisk until well combined. Add oat milk (or other milk), eggs, butter, brown sugar and vanilla; whisk until just combined (some lumps may remain).

2. Coat the waffle iron with cooking spray. Spoon on 1/2 cup batter, spreading it to reach the edges; cook until cooked through and golden brown, 4 to 5 minutes. Repeat with the remaining batter.

3. Top the waffles evenly with berries; serve with maple syrup or yogurt, if desired.

Sweetcorn fritters with eggs & black bean salsa

Ingredients

For the fritters & eggs

- 1 tsp rapeseed oil

- 1 small red onion (85g), finely chopped

- 1 red pepper, deseeded and finely diced

- 100g wholemeal self-raising flour

- 1 tsp smoked paprika

- 1 tsp ground coriander

- 1 tsp baking powder

- 325g can sweetcorn, drained

- 6 large eggs

For the salsa

- 1 small red onion (85g), finely chopped

- 4 tomatoes (320g), chopped

- 2 x 400g cans black beans, drained

- 1 lime, zested and juiced

- ½ x 30g pack coriander, chopped

Instructions

- STEP 1

Heat the oven to 200C/180C fan/gas 6 and line a large baking tray with baking parchment.

- STEP 2

Heat the oil in a small pan and fry the onion and pepper for 5 mins until softened. Meanwhile, mix the flour, spices and baking powder in a bowl. Add the onions, pepper, corn and 2 of the eggs, then mix together well.

• STEP 3

Spoon eight mounds of the mixture onto the baking tray, well-spaced apart, then flatten slightly with the back of the spoon. Bake for 20 mins until set and golden.

• STEP 4

Meanwhile, mix together the salsa Ingredients and poach 2 of the remaining eggs to your liking. Serve the fritters topped with the salsa and the poached eggs.

Nuts & seeds granola

Ingredients

- 150g rolled oats

- 150g mixed nuts (we used whole hazelnuts, flaked almonds and whole pecans)

- 50g mixed seeds (we used a mixed bag containing sunflower, pumpkin, hemp and golden linseed)

- 50g raisins

- 1 tsp ground cinnamon

- ¼ tsp sea salt

- 1 tsp almond extract (vanilla works well too, if you prefer)

- 50ml vegetable oil

- 100ml maple syrup

- milk or yogurt, and fruit (optional), to serve

Instructions

- STEP 1

Heat the oven to 180C/160C fan gas 4. Line a large baking sheet with baking parchment to prevent the granola from sticking. Put all of the dry Ingredients in a large mixing bowl. Whisk together the almond extract, vegetable oil and maple syrup in a jug, then pour into the bowl with the dry Ingredients.

- STEP 2

Mix together well, making sure that all the dry Ingredients are well coated and that there are no dry bits. Tip the mixture onto the lined baking sheet and spread out in an even layer. Cook for about 25-30 mins until golden. You will need to give the mixture a few turns every 8-10 mins to make sure it dries out evenly and doesn't clump together too much. Keep an eye on it as nuts can burn easily.

• STEP 3

Remove from the oven and leave to cool completely on the tray. Break up any large clumps of granola with a wooden spoon. Will keep for up to one month in an airtight container. Serve with milk or yogurt, and fresh seasonal fruit, if you like.

Banana & cinnamon pancakes with blueberry compote

Ingredients

* 65g wholemeal flour

* 1 tsp ground cinnamon, plus extra for sprinkling

* 2 egg, plus 2 egg whites

* 100ml whole milk

* 1 small banana, mashed

* ½ tbsp rapeseed oil

* 320g blueberries

* few mint leaves, to serve

Instructions

* STEP 1

Tip the flour and cinnamon into a bowl, then break in the whole eggs, pour in the milk and whisk together until smooth. Stir in the banana. In a separate bowl, whisk the egg whites until light and fluffy, but not completely stiff, then fold into the pancake mix until evenly incorporated.

• STEP 2

Heat a small amount of oil in a large non-stick frying pan, then add a quarter of the pancake mix, swirl to cover the base of the pan and cook until set and golden. Carefully turn the pancake over with a palette knife and cook the other side. Transfer to a plate, then carry on with the rest of the batter until you have four.

• STEP 3

To make the compote, tip the berries in a non-stick pan and heat gently until the berries just burst but hold their shape. Serve two warm pancakes with half the berries, then scatter with the mint leaves and sprinkle with a little cinnamon. Chill the remaining pancakes and compote and serve the next day. You can reheat them in the microwave or in a pan.

Almond crêpes with avocado & nectarines

Ingredients

- 2 large eggs

- 3 tbsp ground almonds

- 2 tsp rapeseed oil

- 1 avocado, halved, stoned and flesh lightly crushed

- 2 ripe nectarines, stoned and sliced

- seeds from 1/2 pomegranate

- ½ lime, cut into 2 wedges, for squeezing over

Instructions

- STEP 1

Beat one egg and 1 1 /2 tbsp of the almonds in a small bowl with 1 tbsp water. Heat 1 tsp oil in a large non-stick frying pan over a medium heat and pour in the egg mixture, swirling the pan to evenly cover the base. Cook until the mixture sets and turns golden on the underside, about 2 mins. (There is no need to flip it over.) Turn it out onto a plate and make another one with 1 tbsp water, the remaining egg, oil and almonds.

- STEP 2

Top each crêpe with the avocado, nectarines and pomegranate, and squeeze over the lime at the table.

Millet porridge with almond milk & berry compote

Ingredients

- 340g millet

- 1 litre unsweetened fortified almond milk, plus extra to serve

- few mint leaves, to serve

For the compote

- 90g pitted dates, finely chopped

- 500g frozen mixed fruit (ours was a mixed bag of berries, cherries, currants and strawberries)

- 1 cinnamon stick

Instructions

• STEP 1

For the compote, put the dates in a pan with 150ml water, bring to the boil and stir well so they break down. Tip in the frozen fruit and cinnamon stick and cook over a medium heat, stirring every now and then for a couple of minutes. Don't worry about fully thawing larger fruits, as they will defrost in the residual heat and retain their shape in the compote (if you have large strawberries in the mix, you can halve these as they soften). Leave to cool. Will then keep chilled for up to four days.

• STEP 2

Rinse the millet in a sieve, then tip into a deep, heavy-based saucepan and pour in the almond milk and 350ml water. Put over a low heat and once bubbling, leave to simmer for 10-12 mins, stirring frequently until the millet grains are tender, but nutty.

Serve the porridge with the compote. Add a little extra almond milk to serve with a few mint leaves scattered over.

Berry omelette

Ingredients

- 1 large egg

- 1 tbsp skimmed milk

- 3 pinches of cinnamon

- ½ tsp rapeseed oil

- 100g cottage cheese

- 175g chopped strawberry, blueberries and raspberries

Instructions

- STEP 1

Beat egg with milk and cinnamon. Heat oil in a 20cm non-stick frying pan and pour in the egg mixture, swirling to evenly cover the base. Cook for a few mins until set and golden underneath. There's no need to flip it over.

- STEP 2

Place on a plate, spread over cheese, then scatter with berries. Roll up and serve.

LUNCH RECIPES FOR MULTIPLE SCLEROSIS

Sweet Potato & Cauliflower Rice Bowl

Ingredients

• 1 medium sweet potato, peeled if desired, sliced 1/4 inch thick

• 2 teaspoons extra-virgin olive oil plus 2 tablespoons, divided

• 2 pinches salt plus 1/2 teaspoon, divided

• ½ teaspoon ground pepper, divided

• ¼ cup orange juice

• 2 tablespoons lime juice

• ½ cup chopped fresh cilantro, divided

• 3 cloves garlic, minced, divided

• ½ teaspoon ground cumin

• ½ teaspoon dried oregano

• 5 cups cauliflower florets

• 1 (15 ounce) can black beans, rinsed

• 1 firm ripe avocado, sliced

• ½ cup pico de gallo

Directions

1. Preheat oven to 400 degrees F.

2. Toss sweet potato in a medium bowl with 2 teaspoons oil, a pinch of salt and 1/4 teaspoon pepper. Transfer to a baking sheet. Roast until tender, 10 to 14 minutes

3. Meanwhile, combine orange juice, lime juice, 1/4 cup cilantro, 1 minced garlic clove, cumin, oregano and a pinch of salt in a small bowl.

4. Pulse cauliflower florets in two batches in a food processor until chopped into rice-size pieces. Heat the remaining 2 tablespoons oil in a large skillet over medium heat. Add the remaining 2 garlic cloves and cook until fragrant, about 30 seconds. Add the cauliflower rice, the remaining 1/2 teaspoon salt and 1/4 teaspoon pepper; cook, stirring, until softened, 3 to 5 minutes. Remove from heat and stir in the remaining 1/4 cup cilantro.

5. To serve, divide the cauliflower among 4 bowls. Top with the sweet potato, black beans, avocado and pico de gallo. Drizzle each portion with the mojo sauce.

Crispy Chickpea Grain Bowl with Lemon Vinaigrette

Ingredients

- ⅔ cup quinoa

- 1 ⅓ cups water plus 1 tablespoon, divided

- ⅛ teaspoon salt plus 1/4 teaspoon, divided

- 1 (15 ounce) can no-salt-added chickpeas, rinsed

- 1 small red onion, thinly sliced

- 4 teaspoons extra-virgin olive oil plus 2 tablespoons, divided

- ¼ teaspoon ground pepper, divided

• 1 bunch kale, stems removed, thinly sliced (about 5 cups)

• 1 teaspoon Dijon mustard

• 1 clove garlic, minced

• 2 teaspoons lemon zest

• 2 tablespoons lemon juice

• 1 red bell pepper, thinly sliced

• ¼ cup crumbled feta cheese

• 2 tablespoons toasted pumpkin seeds

Directions

1. Preheat oven to 400 degrees F. Coat a large rimmed baking sheet liberally with cooking spray.

2. Combine quinoa, 1 1/3 cups water, and 1/8 teaspoon salt in a medium saucepan. Bring to a boil over medium-high heat. Reduce heat to medium-low, partially cover, and simmer until the quinoa is tender, about 15 minutes. Drain any excess water.

3. Meanwhile, pat chickpeas dry with a paper towel. Toss with onion, 2 teaspoons oil, and 1/8 teaspoon each salt and pepper in a large bowl. Spread out on the prepared baking sheet. Roast for 15 minutes.

4. Toss kale with 2 teaspoons oil and the remaining 1/8 teaspoon salt in the large bowl. Stir the kale into the chickpeas and roast for 15 minutes more.

5. Whisk mustard, garlic, lemon zest, lemon juice, the remaining 1 tablespoon water and the

remaining 1/8 teaspoon pepper in a small bowl. Whisk in the remaining 2 tablespoons oil.

6. Divide the quinoa among 4 serving bowls. Top with the kale mixture, bell pepper slices, feta, and pumpkin seeds. Drizzle with the vinaigrette.

Chicken, Avocado & Quinoa Bowls with Herb Dressing

Ingredients

Roasted Chicken Thighs

- 5 boneless, skinless chicken thighs (about 1 1/4 pounds), trimmed

- ½ teaspoon ground pepper

- ¼ teaspoon salt

Quinoa

- 3 cups low-sodium chicken broth

- 1 tablespoon extra-virgin olive oil

- ¼ teaspoon salt

- 1 ½ cups quinoa

Italian Dressing

- ¾ cup red-wine vinegar

- 5 tablespoons water

- 1 ½ tablespoons sugar

- 1 tablespoon Dijon mustard

- 1 large clove garlic

- 2 teaspoons dried basil

- 2 teaspoons dried oregano

- ½ teaspoon salt

- ½ teaspoon ground pepper

- 1 ¾ cups extra-virgin olive oil

Toppings

- 1 (15 ounce) can chickpeas, rinsed

- 1 avocado, sliced

- 6 radishes, thinly sliced

- 1 cup sprouts or shoots

- ¼ cup toasted seeds or chopped nuts

Directions

1. To prepare chicken: Preheat oven to 425 degrees F. Place chicken on a baking sheet. Sprinkle with 1/2 teaspoon ground pepper and

1/4 teaspoon salt. Roast the chicken until an instant-read thermometer inserted in the thickest part registers 165 degrees F, 14 to 16 minutes. Slice 4 thighs. (Reserve 1 thigh for another use.)

2. Meanwhile, prepare quinoa: Combine broth, 1 tablespoon oil and 1/4 teaspoon salt in a large saucepan. Bring to a simmer over high heat. Stir in quinoa and return to a simmer. Reduce heat and simmer until the quinoa has absorbed all the liquid and the grains have burst, 15 to 20 minutes. Remove from heat, cover and let stand for 5 minutes. (Reserve 2 cups for another use.)

3. To prepare dressing: Combine vinegar, water, sugar, mustard, garlic, basil, oregano, salt and pepper in a blender. Puree until smooth. With the motor running, slowly add oil and puree until creamy. (Transfer 1 3/4 cups to a large mason jar and refrigerate for up to 1 week.)

4. To assemble bowls: Divide 3 cups quinoa among 4 large shallow bowls. Top with the chicken, chickpeas, avocado, radishes and sprouts (or shoots); sprinkle with seeds (or nuts). Drizzle with 3/4 cup dressing.

Black Bean Wraps with Greens & Cilantro Vinaigrette

Ingredients

- 1 cup chopped fresh cilantro

- 3 tablespoons white-wine vinegar

- 2 cloves garlic, peeled

- 1 teaspoon ground cumin, divided

- ½ teaspoon salt, divided

- ¼ cup extra-virgin olive oil

- 3 cups chopped romaine lettuce

- 1 cup chopped radicchio

- 1 cup sliced radishes

- 1 (15 ounce) can no-salt-added black beans, rinsed

- ½ teaspoon chili powder

- ½ teaspoon garlic powder

- 1 ripe avocado

- 1 tablespoon lime juice

- 4 (8 inch) whole-wheat tortillas or wraps

Directions

1. Combine cilantro, vinegar, garlic, 1/2 teaspoon cumin and 1/4 teaspoon salt in a mini food

processor; pulse until finely chopped. With the motor running, slowly stream in oil. Transfer the vinaigrette to a large bowl. Add lettuce, radicchio and radishes and toss to coat.

2. Mash beans, chili powder, garlic powder, the remaining 1/2 teaspoon cumin and 1/4 teaspoon salt in a medium bowl. Mash avocado with lime juice in a small bowl. Spread some of the mashed beans and avocado over each tortilla; top with the salad and roll up.

Veggie & Hummus Sandwich

Ingredients

- 2 slices whole-grain bread

- 3 tablespoons hummus

- ¼ avocado, mashed

- ½ cup mixed salad greens

- ¼ medium red bell pepper, sliced

- ¼ cup sliced cucumber

- ¼ cup shredded carrot

Directions

1. Spread 1 slice of bread with hummus and the other with avocado. Fill the sandwich with greens, bell pepper, cucumber and carrot. Slice in half and serve.

Teriyaki Tofu Rice Bowls

Ingredients

- 2 (10 ounce) package cooked wild rice blend

- 1 tablespoon extra-virgin olive oil

• 1 (18 ounce) package fresh Asian stir-fry vegetables

• 3 tablespoons teriyaki sauce

• 1 (7 ounce) package teriyaki-flavor baked tofu, cubed

Directions

1. Prepare rice according to package Directions. Transfer the rice from the pouches to a shallow bowl to cool.

2. Heat oil in a medium nonstick skillet over medium heat. Add vegetables and sauté until crisp-tender, 4 to 5 minutes. Add teriyaki sauce; toss well to coat the vegetables. Remove from heat; set aside.

3. Divide the cooled rice among 4 single-serving containers. Top each with one-fourth of the

vegetables. Divide tofu among the containers. Seal and refrigerate for up to 4 days. Vent the container and microwave until steaming before serving.

Chickpea Salad Sandwich

Ingredients

• 2 (15.5 ounce) cans no-salt-added chickpeas, rinsed

• 6 tablespoons extra-virgin olive oil

• 3 tablespoons lemon juice

• 2 teaspoons Dijon mustard

• ½ teaspoon garlic powder

• ½ cup finely chopped celery

- ¼ cup finely chopped fresh dill

- ⅛ teaspoon salt

- ⅛ teaspoon ground pepper

- 4 tablespoons vegan mayonnaise

- 8 slices whole-grain bread, toasted

- 4 green lettuce leaves

- 4 thin slices red onion

- 4 tomato slices

Directions

1. Combine chickpeas, oil, lemon juice, mustard and garlic powder in a large bowl. Using a fork or potato masher, crush the chickpeas until most are mashed but some are still whole. Stir in celery, dill, salt and pepper.

2. Spread 1 tablespoon mayonnaise on 1 side of each of 4 slices of bread. Top evenly with lettuce, onion, tomato and chickpea mixture. Top with the remaining 4 slices of bread.

Vegan Grain Bowl

Ingredients

• 1 medium sweet potato, peeled if desired, cut into 1-inch chunks

• 3 tablespoons extra-virgin olive oil, divided

• ½ teaspoon salt, divided

• ½ teaspoon ground pepper, divided

• 2 tablespoons tahini

• 2 tablespoons water

- 1 tablespoon lemon juice

- 1 small clove garlic, minced

- 2 cups cooked quinoa

- 1 15-ounce can chickpeas, rinsed

- 1 firm ripe avocado, diced

- ¼ cup chopped fresh cilantro or parsley

Directions

1. Preheat oven to 425 degrees F.

2. Toss sweet potato with 1 tablespoon oil and 1/4 teaspoon each salt and pepper in a medium bowl. Transfer to a rimmed baking sheet. Roast, stirring once, until tender, 15 to 18 minutes.

3. Meanwhile, whisk the remaining 2 tablespoons oil, tahini, water, lemon juice, garlic and the

remaining 1/4 teaspoon each salt and pepper in a small bowl.

4. To serve, divide quinoa among 4 bowls. Top with equal amounts of sweet potato, chickpeas and avocado. Drizzle with the tahini sauce. Sprinkle with parsley (or cilantro).

Mixed Greens with Lentils & Sliced Apple

Ingredients

- 1 ½ cups mixed salad greens

- ½ cup cooked lentils

- 1 apple, cored and sliced, divided

- 1 ½ tablespoons crumbled feta cheese

- 1 tablespoon red-wine vinegar

- 2 teaspoons extra-virgin olive oil

Directions

1. Top greens with lentils, about half the apple slices and the feta. Drizzle with vinegar and oil. Serve with the remaining apple slices on the side.

Meal-Prep Roasted Vegetable Bowls with Pesto

Ingredients

- 3 tablespoons extra-virgin olive oil, divided

- ½ teaspoon garlic powder

- ¼ teaspoon salt

- ¼ teaspoon ground pepper

- 4 cups broccoli florets

- 2 medium red bell peppers, quartered

- 1 cup sliced red onion

- 3 cups cooked brown rice

- 1 (15 ounce) can chickpeas, rinsed

- 4 tablespoons prepared pesto

Directions

1. Preheat oven to 450 degrees F.

2. Whisk 2 tablespoons oil, garlic powder, salt and pepper together in a large bowl. Add broccoli, peppers and onion; toss to coat. Transfer to a large rimmed baking sheet and roast, stirring once, until the vegetables are tender, about 20 minutes. Chop the peppers when cool enough to handle.

3. Stir the remaining 1 tablespoon oil into rice. Place about 3/4 cup of the rice in each of four 2-cup microwave-safe, lidded containers. Divide chickpeas and the roasted vegetables among the bowls. Top each with 1 tablespoon pesto.

4. To reheat: Microwave each container on High until heated through, 1 to 2 minutes.

White Bean & Avocado Sandwich

Ingredients

- 2 medium avocados

- 1 (15 ounce) can white beans, rinsed

- 2 tablespoons lemon juice

- 1 tablespoon extra-virgin olive oil

- 1 clove garlic, grated

- ¼ teaspoon chopped fresh thyme

- ¼ teaspoon ground pepper

- 8 slices whole-wheat bread, toasted

- 1 cup chopped jarred roasted red peppers, rinsed

- 8 thin slices sharp Cheddar cheese (about 4 ounces)

- 4 cups baby lettuce

Directions

1. Mash avocados, beans, lemon juice, oil, garlic, thyme and pepper in a medium bowl until well combined but still slightly chunky. Divide among 4 slices of bread (1/2 cup each). Top each sandwich with 1/4 cup red peppers, 2 slices cheese, 1 cup lettuce and the remaining bread.

Quinoa, Avocado & Chickpea Salad over Mixed Greens

Ingredients

- ⅔ cup water

- ⅓ cup quinoa

- ¼ teaspoon kosher salt or other coarse salt

- 1 clove garlic, crushed and peeled

- 2 teaspoons grated lemon zest

- 3 tablespoons lemon juice

- 3 tablespoons olive oil

- ¼ teaspoon ground pepper

- 1 cup rinsed no-salt-added canned chickpeas

- 1 medium carrot, shredded (1/2 cup)

- ½ avocado, diced

- 1 (5 ounce) package prewashed mixed greens, such as spring mix or baby kale-spinach blend (8 cups packed)

Directions

1. Bring water to a boil in a small saucepan. Stir in quinoa. Reduce heat to low, cover, and simmer until all the liquid is absorbed, about 15 minutes. Use a fork to fluff and separate the grains; let cool for 5 minutes.

2. Meanwhile, sprinkle salt over garlic on a cutting board. Mash the garlic with the side of a spoon until a paste forms. Scrape into a medium bowl. Whisk in lemon zest, lemon juice, oil, and

pepper. Transfer 3 Tbsp. of the dressing to a small bowl and set aside.

3. Add chickpeas, carrot, and avocado to the bowl with the remaining dressing; gently toss to combine. Let stand for 5 minutes to allow flavors to blend. Add the quinoa and gently toss to coat.

4. Place greens in a large bowl and toss with the reserved 3 Tbsp. dressing. Divide the greens between 2 plates and top with the quinoa mixture.

Tips

To make ahead: Prepare quinoa (Step 1) and refrigerate for up to 2 days.

Avocado Toast with Burrata

Ingredients

- 1 slice whole-grain toast (3/4 inch thick)

- ½ large ripe avocado, thinly sliced

- 1 teaspoon lemon juice

- ⅛ teaspoon kosher salt

- ⅛ teaspoon ground pepper

- 1 ½ ounces burrata or fresh mozzarella cheese

- 1 teaspoon finely sliced fresh basil

- 1 teaspoon minced fresh chives

- Pinch of Aleppo pepper

Directions

1. Top toast with avocado. Drizzle with lemon juice and sprinkle with salt and pepper. Top with

burrata (or mozzarella), basil, chives and Aleppo pepper.

Green Goddess Salad

Ingredients

• ½ avocado, peeled and pitted

• ¾ cup nonfat buttermilk

• 2 tablespoons chopped fresh herbs, such as tarragon, sorrel and/or chives

• 2 teaspoons tarragon vinegar, or white-wine vinegar

• 1 teaspoon anchovy paste, or minced anchovy fillet

• 8 cups bite-size pieces green leaf lettuce

- 12 ounces peeled and deveined cooked shrimp, (21-25 per pound; see Ingredient note)

- ½ cucumber, sliced

- 1 cup cherry or grape tomatoes

- 1 cup canned chickpeas, rinsed

- 1 cup rinsed and chopped canned artichoke hearts

- ½ cup chopped celery

Directions

1. Puree avocado, buttermilk, herbs, vinegar and anchovy in a blender until smooth.

2. Divide lettuce among 4 plates. Top with shrimp, cucumber, tomatoes, chickpeas, artichoke hearts and celery. Drizzle the dressing over the salads.

Stuffed Sweet Potato with Hummus Dressing

Ingredients

- 1 large sweet potato, scrubbed

- ¾ cup chopped kale

- 1 cup canned black beans, rinsed

- ¼ cup hummus

- 2 tablespoons water

Directions

1. Prick sweet potato all over with a fork. Microwave on High until cooked through, 7 to 10 minutes.

2. Meanwhile, wash kale and drain, allowing water to cling to the leaves. Place in a medium

saucepan; cover and cook over medium-high heat, stirring once or twice, until wilted. Add beans; add a tablespoon or two of water if the pot is dry. Continue cooking, uncovered, stirring occasionally, until the mixture is steaming hot, 1 to 2 minutes.

3. Split the sweet potato open and top with the kale and bean mixture. Combine hummus and 2 tablespoons water in a small dish. Add additional water as needed to reach desired consistency. Drizzle the hummus dressing over the stuffed sweet potato.

Orzo Salad with Chickpeas & Artichoke Hearts

Ingredients

• 1/2 cup orzo, or other tiny pasta

- 1 ½ teaspoons extra-virgin olive oil

- 1 clove garlic, crushed and peeled

- ⅛ teaspoon salt

- 1 ½ tablespoons lemon juice

- ⅛ teaspoon freshly ground pepper

- 1 14-ounce can artichoke hearts, drained and chopped

- 1 7-ounce can chickpeas, rinsed

- ⅓ cup crumbled feta cheese

- 2 tablespoons chopped fresh dill

- 1 ½ tablespoons chopped fresh mint

- 1 large tomato, chopped

- 2 cups baby spinach leaves

Directions

1. Bring a small saucepan of water to a boil. Cook orzo until just tender, about 9 minutes, or according to package **Directions**. Drain and rinse under cold water until cool. Press to remove excess water. Transfer to a medium bowl and toss with oil.

2. Mash garlic and salt into a paste with the back of a spoon in a medium bowl. Whisk in lemon juice and pepper. Add the cooked orzo, artichokes, chickpeas, feta, dill and mint; toss gently to combine. Add tomatoes and toss again.

3. Divide spinach between 2 plates and top with the salad.

Tips

Make Ahead **Tip**: Prepare the salad--without the tomatoes and spinach--cover and refrigerate for up to 1 day. Add the tomatoes just before serving and serve over the spinach.

Avocado Tuna Spinach Salad

Ingredients

- ½ (5 ounce) can water-packed tuna

- ¼ cup diced avocado

- ¼ cup halved cherry tomatoes

- 1 ½ tablespoons poppy seed dressing

- 1 tablespoon diced red onion

- 1 tablespoon extra-virgin olive oil

- 2 cups baby spinach

• 1 tablespoon sunflower seeds

Directions

1. Combine tuna, avocado, tomatoes, dressing, onion and oil in a medium bowl. Serve over spinach and sprinkle with sunflower seeds.

White Bean & Veggie Salad

Ingredients

• 2 cups mixed salad greens

• ¾ cup veggies of your choice, such as chopped cucumbers and cherry tomatoes

• ⅓ cup canned white beans, rinsed and drained

• ½ avocado, diced

• 1 tablespoon red-wine vinegar

- 2 teaspoons extra-virgin olive oil

- ¼ teaspoon kosher salt

- Freshly ground pepper to taste

Directions

1. Combine greens, veggies, beans and avocado in a medium bowl. Drizzle with vinegar and oil and season with salt and pepper. Toss to combine and transfer to a large plate.

Black Bean-Quinoa Bowl

Ingredients

- ¾ cup canned black beans, rinsed

- ⅔ cup cooked quinoa

- ¼ cup hummus

- 1 tablespoon lime juice

- ¼ medium avocado, diced

- 3 tablespoons pico de gallo

- 2 tablespoons chopped fresh cilantro

Directions

1. Combine beans and quinoa in a bowl. Stir hummus and lime juice together in a small bowl; thin with water to desired consistency. Drizzle the hummus dressing over the beans and quinoa. Top with avocado, pico de gallo and cilantro.

Lemony Lentil Salad with Feta

Ingredients

- ⅓ cup lemon juice

- ⅓ cup chopped fresh dill

- 2 teaspoons Dijon mustard

- ¼ teaspoon salt, or to taste

- ⅓ cup extra-virgin olive oil

- Freshly ground pepper, to taste

- 2 15-ounce cans lentils, rinsed, or 3 cups cooked brown or green lentils

- 1 cup crumbled feta cheese, (about 4 ounces)

- 1 medium red bell pepper, seeded and diced (about 1 cup)

- 1 cup diced seedless cucumber

- ½ cup finely chopped red onion

Directions

1. Whisk lemon juice, dill, mustard, salt and pepper in a large bowl. Gradually whisk in oil. Add lentils, feta, bell pepper, cucumber and onion; toss to coat.

Tips

Make Ahead Tip: The salad will keep, covered, in the refrigerator for up to 8 hours.

DINNER RECIPES FOR MULTIPLE SCLEROSIS

Sweet Potato & Cauliflower Rice Bowl

Ingredients

• 1 medium sweet potato, peeled if desired, sliced 1/4 inch thick

• 2 teaspoons extra-virgin olive oil plus 2 tablespoons, divided

• 2 pinches salt plus 1/2 teaspoon, divided

• ½ teaspoon ground pepper, divided

• ¼ cup orange juice

• 2 tablespoons lime juice

• ½ cup chopped fresh cilantro, divided

- 3 cloves garlic, minced, divided

- ½ teaspoon ground cumin

- ½ teaspoon dried oregano

- 5 cups cauliflower florets

- 1 (15 ounce) can black beans, rinsed

- 1 firm ripe avocado, sliced

- ½ cup pico de gallo

Directions

1. Preheat oven to 400 degrees F.

2. Toss sweet potato in a medium bowl with 2 teaspoons oil, a pinch of salt and 1/4 teaspoon pepper. Transfer to a baking sheet. Roast until tender, 10 to 14 minutes

3. Meanwhile, combine orange juice, lime juice, 1/4 cup cilantro, 1 minced garlic clove, cumin, oregano and a pinch of salt in a small bowl.

4. Pulse cauliflower florets in two batches in a food processor until chopped into rice-size pieces. Heat the remaining 2 tablespoons oil in a large skillet over medium heat. Add the remaining 2 garlic cloves and cook until fragrant, about 30 seconds. Add the cauliflower rice, the remaining 1/2 teaspoon salt and 1/4 teaspoon pepper; cook, stirring, until softened, 3 to 5 minutes. Remove from heat and stir in the remaining 1/4 cup cilantro.

5. To serve, divide the cauliflower among 4 bowls. Top with the sweet potato, black beans, avocado and pico de gallo. Drizzle each portion with the mojo sauce.

Butternut Squash Soup with Apple Grilled Cheese Sandwiches

Ingredients

• 2 tablespoons grapeseed oil or coconut oil, divided

• 1 cup chopped onion

• 2 tablespoons minced fresh ginger

• 1 teaspoon ground cumin

• 1 teaspoon ground turmeric

• ¼ teaspoon cayenne pepper, plus more for garnish

• 5 cups cubed (1-inch) peeled butternut squash

• 1 (15 ounce) can light coconut milk, divided

- 2 cups low-sodium no-chicken broth or chicken broth

- 1 small apple, thinly sliced, divided

- ¾ teaspoon salt

- 1 tablespoon lime juice

- 4 slices whole-wheat country bread

- 1 cup shredded smoked Gouda or Cheddar cheese

- Ground pepper for garnish

Directions

1. Heat 1 tablespoon oil in a large saucepan over medium heat. Add onion and ginger; cook, stirring, until starting to soften, about 3 minutes. Add cumin, turmeric and cayenne; cook, stirring, for 30 seconds. Add squash, coconut milk

(reserve 4 tablespoons for garnish, if desired), broth, half the apple slices and salt. Bring to a boil. Reduce the heat to maintain a simmer and cook, stirring occasionally, until the squash is tender, about 20 minutes. Stir in lime juice. Remove from heat.

2. Puree the soup in the pan using an immersion blender or in batches in a blender. (Use caution when blending hot liquids.)

3. Divide 1/2 cup cheese between 2 slices of bread. Top with the remaining apple slices, cheese and bread. Heat the remaining 1 tablespoon oil in a large nonstick skillet over medium heat. Add the sandwiches and cook until lightly browned on both sides and the cheese is melted, about 2 minutes per side. Cut in half. Garnish the soup with the reserved coconut milk, more cayenne and ground pepper, if desired.

Honey-Mustard Pork with Spinach & Smashed White Beans

Ingredients

- 1 ¼ pounds pork tenderloin, trimmed

- ½ teaspoon salt, divided

- ½ teaspoon ground pepper

- 3 tablespoons extra-virgin olive oil, divided

- 1 pound mature spinach, chopped

- 2 cloves garlic, minced

- 1 ½ teaspoons chopped fresh sage

- ¼ teaspoon crushed red pepper

- 2 (15 ounce) cans low-sodium cannellini beans, rinsed

- ¾ cup low-sodium chicken broth, divided

- 3 tablespoons honey

- 2 tablespoons whole-grain mustard

Directions

1. Preheat oven to 425 degrees F.

2. Season pork with 1/4 teaspoon salt and pepper. Heat 1 tablespoon oil in a large ovenproof skillet over medium-high heat. Add pork and cook, turning often, until browned on all sides, 3 to 5 minutes total. Transfer the pan to the oven. Roast until an instant-read thermometer inserted in the center registers 145 degrees F, 12 to 15 minutes.

3. Meanwhile, heat 1 tablespoon oil in a large pot over medium-high heat. Add spinach and 1/8

teaspoon salt; cook, stirring, until wilted, 2 to 3 minutes. Transfer to a bowl; cover to keep warm.

4. Heat the remaining 1 tablespoon oil in the pot over medium heat. Add garlic, sage and crushed red pepper; cook for 30 seconds. Add beans, 1/2 cup broth and the remaining 1/8 teaspoon salt. Mash with a potato masher until almost smooth. Reduce heat and cook, stirring often, until hot, about 5 minutes. Remove from heat and cover.

5. Transfer the pork to a clean cutting board and let rest for 5 minutes. Add honey, mustard and the remaining 1/4 cup broth to the pan (the handle will be hot). Bring to a boil over medium-high heat, scraping up any browned bits. Reduce heat and simmer until thickened slightly, 1 to 2 minutes.

6. Slice the pork. Serve with the spinach, mashed beans and sauce.

Scallion-Ginger Beef & Broccoli

Ingredients

- ⅓ cup reduced-sodium tamari or soy sauce

- ¼ cup low-sodium chicken broth

- 2 tablespoons brown sugar

- 2 tablespoons cornstarch, divided

- 1 pound sirloin steak, thinly sliced

- 3 tablespoons peanut or canola oil, divided

- 6 cups broccoli florets

- ½ cup sliced scallions, plus more for garnish

- 1 tablespoon finely grated ginger

- 1 teaspoon finely grated garlic

- 2 cups cooked brown rice

- Crushed red pepper for garnish

Directions

1. Whisk tamari (or soy sauce), broth, brown sugar and 1 tablespoon cornstarch in a small bowl. Toss steak with the remaining 1 tablespoon cornstarch.

2. Heat 2 tablespoons oil in a large flat-bottom wok or cast-iron skillet over medium-high heat. Add the steak and cook, stirring once, until browned, about 4 minutes. Transfer to a clean plate. Add the remaining 1 tablespoon oil and broccoli; cook, stirring occasionally, until slightly tender, about 2 minutes. Stir in scallions, ginger

and garlic; cook, stirring, until fragrant, about 30 seconds. Whisk the tamari mixture and add it, along with the beef, back to the pan; cook until the sauce thickens, about 1 minute. Serve over brown rice and garnish with crushed red pepper, if desired.

Sheet-Pan Maple-Mustard Pork Chops & Carrots

Ingredients

- 4 tablespoons extra-virgin olive oil, divided

- 1 tablespoon whole-grain mustard

- 1 tablespoon maple syrup

- 4 (5 ounce) bone-in, center-cut pork chops (1/2 inch thick)

- 1 ½ pounds rainbow carrots, cut diagonally into 1/4-inch slices

- 2 teaspoons finely chopped garlic

- 1 teaspoon coarsely chopped peeled fresh ginger

- ½ teaspoon ground turmeric

- ¾ teaspoon kosher salt

- ¾ teaspoon ground pepper

- ¼ cup chopped flat-leaf parsley

Directions

1. Position a rack in the lower third of the oven and preheat to 450 degrees F.

2. Whisk 1 tablespoon oil, mustard and maple syrup in a small bowl. Place pork chops on one

side of a rimmed baking sheet. Brush the tops with the oil mixture. Place carrots on the other side and drizzle with the remaining 3 tablespoons oil. Sprinkle garlic, ginger and turmeric on the carrots and toss to coat. Season everything with salt and pepper. Roast for 10 minutes.

3. Turn broiler to high. Broil until an instant-read thermometer inserted in the thickest part of a chop without touching the bone registers 145 degrees F, about 4 minutes. Continue cooking the carrots, if needed, until tender and glazed, 2 to 5 minutes more. Serve sprinkled with parsley.

Golden Vegetable Soup

Ingredients

• 2 tablespoons extra-virgin olive oil

- 1 medium yellow onion, chopped

- 1 medium butternut squash, peeled and cut into 1-inch pieces (about 6 cups)

- 1 small serrano pepper, seeded and chopped

- 1 tablespoon minced fresh ginger

- 1 teaspoon ground coriander

- 1 teaspoon ground cumin

- ½ teaspoon ground turmeric

- ¾ teaspoon toasted fennel seeds, divided

- 2 cups cauliflower florets

- 4 cups reduced-sodium vegetable broth

- 1 ¼ cups well-shaken light coconut milk, divided

- 1 ½ teaspoons lime juice

- ½ teaspoon salt

Directions

1. Heat oil in a large Dutch oven or heavy stockpot over medium heat. Add onion and squash; cook, stirring often, until the onion is translucent, about 7 minutes. Add serrano and ginger; cook, stirring often, until fragrant, about 1 minute.

2. Reduce heat to medium-low and add coriander, cumin, turmeric and 1/4 teaspoon fennel seeds. Cook, stirring constantly, until fragrant, about 1 minute. Stir in cauliflower and broth. Bring to a boil over medium-high heat; reduce heat to medium-low, and simmer, stirring occasionally, until the squash is fork-tender, 25 to 30 minutes.

3. Working in 2 batches, transfer the squash mixture to a blender. Secure the lid on the blender and remove the center piece to allow steam to escape. Place a clean towel over the opening. Process until smooth, about 1 minute. (Use caution when pureeing hot liquids.) Return the mixture to the pot.

4. Stir 1 cup coconut milk into the soup. Bring to a gentle simmer over medium-low heat. Stir in lime juice and salt. Remove from heat.

5. Divide the soup among 4 bowls. Top each with 1 tablespoon coconut milk and a pinch of fennel seeds.

Ginger-Tahini Oven-Baked Salmon & Vegetables

Ingredients

- 1 large sweet potato, cubed (about 12 oz.)

- 1 pound white button or cremini mushrooms, cut into 1-inch pieces (6 cups)

- 2 tablespoons olive oil, divided

- ½ teaspoon salt, divided

- 1 pound green beans, trimmed

- 2 tablespoons reduced-sodium soy sauce

- 1 tablespoon plus 2 tsp. tahini

- 1 tablespoon plus 1 tsp. honey

- 1 ½ teaspoons finely grated fresh ginger

- 1 ¼ pounds salmon, preferably wild-caught, cut into 4 portions

- 2 teaspoons rice vinegar

- 2 tablespoons chopped fresh chives (Optional)

Directions

1. Place a large rimmed baking sheet in the oven. Position one rack in the middle of the oven and another about 6 inches from the broiler. Preheat to 425 degrees F.

2. Combine sweet potato, mushrooms, 1 Tbsp. oil, and 1/4 tsp. salt in a large bowl; toss to coat.

3. Remove the baking sheet from the oven. Spread the vegetable mixture in an even layer on the pan; roast, stirring once, until the sweet potatoes are starting to brown, about 20 minutes.

4. Meanwhile, toss green beans with the remaining 1 Tbsp. oil and 1/4 tsp. salt. Combine soy sauce, tahini, honey, and ginger in a small bowl.

5. Remove the pan from the oven. Move the mushrooms and sweet potatoes to one side and place the green beans on the other side. Place salmon in the middle, nestling it on top of the vegetables, if necessary. Spread half of the tahini sauce on top of the salmon. Roast until the salmon flakes, 8 to 10 minutes more. Turn broiler to high; move the pan to the top rack and broil until the salmon is glazed, about 3 minutes.

6. Stir vinegar into the remaining tahini sauce and drizzle it over the salmon and vegetables. Garnish with chives, if desired, and serve.

Tips

To make ahead: Prepare tahini sauce (Step 4) up to 1 day ahead; cover and refrigerate.

Apple-Cranberry Spinach Salad with Goat Cheese

Ingredients

- 3 tablespoons apple cider vinegar

- 4 teaspoons spicy brown mustard

- 4 teaspoons pure maple syrup

- 1 tablespoon minced shallot (from 1 small shallot)

- ½ teaspoon kosher salt

- ½ teaspoon black pepper

- 3 tablespoons extra-virgin olive oil

- 1 (10 ounce) package fresh baby spinach

- 2 large Pink Lady apples, thinly sliced

- ½ cup sweetened dried cranberries

- ½ cup chopped toasted pecans, divided

- 2 ½ ounces semi-soft goat cheese, crumbled (about 1/3 cup)

Directions

1. Whisk together vinegar, mustard, syrup, shallot, salt and pepper in a small bowl; slowly whisk in olive oil until completely blended.

2. Toss together spinach, apples, dried cranberries, half of the pecans and dressing in a large bowl. Transfer to a serving platter and sprinkle with goat cheese and remaining pecans. Serve immediately.

Vegan Pumpkin Soup

Ingredients

- 2 tablespoons extra-virgin olive oil

- 1 cup chopped yellow onion

- 1 cup chopped celery

- 1 tablespoon minced garlic

- 1 teaspoon ground turmeric

- 1 teaspoon ground cumin

- ½ teaspoon ground ginger

- ½ teaspoon ground pepper

- 1 (15 ounce) can unseasoned pumpkin puree

- 3 cups reduced-sodium vegetable broth

- ½ teaspoon salt

- ¾ cup coarsely chopped unsalted roasted cashews, divided

- ¼ cup chopped scallions

- ½ teaspoon smoked paprika

Directions

1. Heat oil in a large saucepan over medium-high heat. Add onion and celery; cook, stirring occasionally, until softened, about 7 minutes. Add garlic, turmeric, cumin, ginger and pepper; cook, stirring constantly, until fragrant, about 1 minute. Add pumpkin, broth, salt and 1/2 cup cashews. Bring to a boil over high heat. Reduce heat to medium-low to maintain a simmer; cover and simmer until the vegetables are tender and the cashews are soft, about 15 minutes.

2. Pour the soup into a blender. Secure the lid on the blender and remove the center piece to allow steam to escape. Place a clean towel over the opening. Process until smooth, about 30 seconds (use caution when blending hot liquids). (Alternatively, process the soup in the pot using an immersion blender on high speed for 1 to 2 minutes.) Ladle the soup evenly into 4 bowls (or pumpkins, see Tip); sprinkle with scallions, paprika and the remaining 1/4 cup cashews.

Tips

Tip: To make Pumpkin Soup Bowls: Preheat oven to 350 degrees F. Cut off and discard tops from 4 small pumpkins (pie pumpkins work well). Scoop out and discard pulp and seeds, removing as much pulp as possible. Brush the pumpkin insides with a little olive oil and, if desired, sprinkle with salt and pepper. Arrange the pumpkins, cut-sides up, on a baking sheet. Bake until the inside flesh is tender when pierced with a fork, 20 to 30 minutes. Let cool slightly before filling with soup.

Delicata Squash & Tofu Curry

Ingredients

• 2 tablespoons curry powder, preferably Madras

• ½ teaspoon salt

• ¼ teaspoon freshly ground pepper

• 1 14-ounce package extra-firm or firm water-packed tofu

• 4 teaspoons canola oil, divided

• 1 large delicata squash (about 1 pound), halved, seeded and cut into 1-inch cubes

• 1 medium onion, halved and sliced

• 2 teaspoons grated fresh ginger

• 1 14-ounce can "lite" coconut milk

• 1 teaspoon light brown sugar

• 8 cups coarsely chopped kale or chard, tough stems removed

• 1 tablespoon lime juice, plus more to taste

Directions

1. Combine curry powder, salt and pepper in a small bowl. Blot tofu dry with a paper towel and cut into 1-inch cubes; toss the tofu in a medium bowl with 1 teaspoon of the spice mixture.

2. Heat 2 teaspoons oil in a large nonstick skillet over medium-high heat. Add the tofu and cook,

stirring every 2 minutes, until browned, 6 to 8 minutes total. Transfer to a plate.

3. Heat the remaining 2 teaspoons oil over medium-high heat. Add squash, onion, ginger and the remaining spice mixture; cook, stirring, until the vegetables are lightly browned, 4 to 5 minutes. Add coconut milk and brown sugar; bring to a boil. Add half the kale (or chard) and cook, stirring, until slightly wilted, about 1 minute. Stir in the rest of the greens and cook, stirring, for 1 minute. Return the tofu to the pan, cover and cook, stirring once or twice, until the squash and greens are tender, 3 to 5 minutes more. Remove from the heat and stir in lime juice.

Ginger Beef Stir-Fry with Peppers

Ingredients

* 12 ounces lean flank steak, trimmed

* 1 ½ teaspoon cornstarch

* 1 tablespoon reduced-sodium soy sauce, divided

* 1 teaspoon dry sherry plus 1 Tbsp., divided

* 1 teaspoon vegetable oil plus 1 Tbsp., divided

* 4 teaspoon hoisin sauce

* 4 teaspoon ketchup

* 1 - 3 teaspoons chile-garlic sauce or Sriracha

* 3 slices peeled ginger, smashed

* 1 small yellow onion, thinly sliced

* 1 cup diced green bell pepper (1-inch)

* 1 cup diced red bell pepper (1-inch)

• 2 tablespoons unsalted beef broth

Directions

1. Cut beef with the grain into 2-inch-wide strips. Cut each strip across the grain into 1/4-inch-thick slices. Combine the beef, cornstarch, 1½ tsp. soy sauce, and 1 tsp. sherry in a medium bowl; stir until the cornstarch is no longer visible. Add 1 tsp. oil and stir until the beef is lightly coated.

2. Combine hoisin sauce, ketchup, chile-garlic sauce (or Sriracha) to taste, and the remaining 1½ tsp. soy sauce and 1 Tbsp. sherry in a small bowl. Set aside.

3. Heat a 14-inch flat-bottomed carbon-steel wok (or a 12-inch stainless-steel skillet) over high heat until a drop of water vaporizes within 1 to 2 seconds of contact. Swirl in the remaining 1 Tbsp. oil. Add ginger and stir-fry until fragrant, about

10 seconds. Push the ginger to the sides of the pan and add the beef in an even layer. Cook, undisturbed, until the beef begins to brown, about 1 minute. Add onion and, using a metal spatula, stir-fry until the beef is lightly browned but not cooked through, 30 seconds to 1 minute more. Transfer the beef and onion mixture to a plate.

4. Add green and red peppers and broth to the pan. Cover and cook over high heat until the peppers are bright green and red and almost all the liquid has been absorbed, about 1 minute. Return the beef and onion and any accumulated juices to the pan. Add the reserved sauce and stir-fry until the beef is just cooked through and the peppers are tender-crisp, 30 seconds to 1 minute. Remove the ginger, if desired.

Tinola (Filipino Ginger-Garlic Chicken Soup)

Ingredients

- 3 tablespoons canola oil or avocado oil

- ½ cup chopped yellow onion

- ¼ cup thinly sliced fresh ginger

- 6 cloves garlic, minced

- 1 pound boneless, skinless chicken thighs, trimmed and cut into 1/2-inch pieces

- 4 cups low-sodium chicken broth

- 1 ½ cups peeled and cubed green papaya or chayote

* 2 cups chopped malunggay leaves or bok choy leaves

* 1 tablespoon fish sauce

* ¼ teaspoon salt

* ¼ teaspoon ground black pepper

Directions

1. Heat oil in a large pot over medium heat. Add onion, ginger and garlic; cook, stirring, until the onion starts to turn translucent, about 3 minutes. Add chicken and broth; cook, stirring, until the chicken is just cooked through, about 5 minutes. Add papaya (or chayote), malunggay (or bok choy), fish sauce, salt and pepper; continue simmering until the vegetables are tender and the flavors have melded, about 5 minutes more.

Mixed Greens with Lentils & Sliced Apple

Ingredients

- 1 ½ cups mixed salad greens

- ½ cup cooked lentils

- 1 apple, cored and sliced, divided

- 1 ½ tablespoons crumbled feta cheese

- 1 tablespoon red-wine vinegar

- 2 teaspoons extra-virgin olive oil

Directions

1. Top greens with lentils, about half the apple slices and the feta. Drizzle with vinegar and oil. Serve with the remaining apple slices on the side.

Lamb & Beef Balti

Ingredients

- 1 ½ cups water

- 1 cup brown basmati rice

- 8 ounces lean ground beef

- 8 ounces ground lamb

- 3 cups chopped yellow onions

- 2 tablespoons chopped garlic

- 1 tablespoon ground turmeric (see Tip)

- 2 teaspoons grated fresh ginger

- 1 ½ teaspoons ground coriander

- 1 teaspoon ground cumin

- 3 tablespoons tomato paste

- 3 cups unsalted beef broth

- 2 tablespoons Worcestershire sauce

- ¾ teaspoon salt

- ¼ cup low-fat plain Greek yogurt

- 3 tablespoons chopped fresh cilantro

Directions

1. Combine water and rice in a medium saucepan; bring to a boil over high heat. Reduce heat to a simmer, cover and cook until the water is absorbed, about 40 minutes.

2. Meanwhile, cook beef and lamb in a large skillet over medium-high heat, crumbling with a wooden spoon, until no longer pink, 5 to 6

minutes. Add onions and cook, stirring occasionally, until translucent, 6 to 8 minutes.

3. Increase heat to high. Add garlic, turmeric, ginger, coriander and cumin; cook, stirring, until fragrant, about 1 minute. Stir in tomato paste and cook, stirring, for 1 minute. Stir in broth, Worcestershire and salt; bring to a boil. Reduce heat to medium and simmer, stirring occasionally, until thickened, 13 to 15 minutes.

4. Serve the balti over the rice, topped with some yogurt and cilantro with naan bread on the side.

Tips

To make ahead: Refrigerate balti (Steps 2-3) for up to 3 days.

Tip: Turmeric has anti-inflammatory properties. Researchers found that just 2 grams (the amount in one serving of this dish) can reduce muscle soreness after an intense workout.

Curried Parsnip & Apple Soup

Ingredients

• 1 tablespoon extra-virgin olive oil

• 1 ½ pounds parsnips (about 5 medium), peeled, cored and chopped

• 1 large onion, finely chopped

• 3 medium cloves garlic, finely chopped

• 4 cups low-sodium chicken broth

• 1 cup water

• 1 medium russet potato (about 8 ounces), peeled and chopped

- 1 large Granny Smith apple, peeled and chopped

- 1 ½ teaspoons mild curry powder

- 1 ½ teaspoons ground coriander, plus more for garnish

- 1 teaspoon ground cumin

- ½ teaspoon ground ginger

- 4 teaspoons lemon juice

- ½ teaspoon salt

- ¼ teaspoon freshly ground pepper

- ½ cup low-fat plain yogurt

Directions

1. Heat oil in a large pot over medium-high heat. Add parsnips and onion and cook, stirring occasionally, until the onion begins to brown, 5 to 7 minutes. Add garlic and cook, stirring occasionally, until fragrant, 45 seconds. Add broth, water, potato, apple, curry powder, coriander, cumin and ginger; bring to a boil. Cover, reduce heat to medium-low and simmer until the vegetables are tender when mashed against the side of the pot with a wooden spoon, about 20 minutes.

2. Puree the soup in the pot with an immersion blender until smooth. (Alternatively, blend the soup in batches in a blender with the lid slightly ajar. Use caution when blending hot liquids. Return the soup to the pot.) Add lemon juice, salt and pepper. Serve with dollops of yogurt swirled on top, garnished with pinches of coriander.

Loaded Chicken-Quinoa Salad

Ingredients

- ¾ cup shredded cooked chicken breast

- ½ cup cooked quinoa

- 1 cup roasted root vegetables

- 1-2 tablespoons vinaigrette

- ¼ avocado, sliced

- 1 tablespoon crumbled feta cheese

- 1 tablespoon sunflower seeds

Directions

1. Combine chicken, quinoa and roasted vegetables in a bowl; drizzle with vinaigrette. Top with avocado, feta and sunflower seeds.

Roasted Carrot Soup

Ingredients

• 1 ½ pounds carrots, peeled and cut into 2- to 3-inch pieces

• 1 onion, peeled and quartered

• 3 cloves garlic, unpeeled

• 1 (1 inch) piece fresh ginger, peeled and sliced

• 1 tablespoon olive oil

• 2 cups unsweetened almond milk

• 1 cup low-sodium chicken broth

• 1 teaspoon coarsely ground black pepper

• 1 cup water

• 1 teaspoon Shredded carrot

• 1 Fresh basil leaves

Directions

1. Preheat oven to 400 degrees F. In a large bowl, combine the carrot pieces, the onion, garlic, and ginger. Drizzle with olive oil; toss to coat. Arrange vegetables in a single layer on a 15x10x1-inch baking pan. Bake 50 to 60 minutes or until carrots are very tender. Cool slightly.

2. Squeeze garlic cloves from their skins into a food processor or blender. Add roasted carrots, onion, and ginger; cover and process or blend with several on/off turns until the vegetables are chopped. Add almond milk, broth, and pepper. Cover and process or blend until smooth.

3. Transfer to a medium saucepan. Stir in the water. Cook and stir until heated through. If desired, garnish with shredded carrot and basil leaves.

Beef Stir-Fry with Baby Bok Choy & Ginger

Ingredients

• 12 ounces beef flank steak, trimmed

• 1 tablespoon minced fresh ginger

• 1 ½ teaspoons reduced-sodium soy sauce

• 1 teaspoon dry sherry plus 1 Tbsp., divided

• 1 teaspoon cornstarch

• 1 teaspoon toasted sesame oil

• 2 tablespoons oyster-flavored sauce, preferably Lee Kum Kee Premium

• 1 tablespoon vegetable oil

• 1 pound baby bok choy, trimmed and cut into 2-inch pieces (about 8 cups)

• 3 tablespoons unsalted chicken broth

Directions

1. Cut beef with the grain into 2-inch-wide strips. Cut each strip across the grain into 1/4-inch-thick slices. Combine the beef, ginger, soy sauce, 1 tsp. sherry, and cornstarch in a medium bowl; stir until the cornstarch is no longer visible. Add sesame oil and stir until the beef is lightly coated.

2. Combine oyster-flavored sauce and the remaining 1 Tbsp. sherry in a small bowl. Set aside.

3. Heat a 14-inch flat-bottomed carbon-steel wok (or a 12-inch stainless-steel skillet) over high heat until a drop of water vaporizes within 1 to 2 seconds of contact. Swirl in vegetable oil. Add the beef in an even layer; cook, undisturbed, until it begins to brown, about 1 minute. Using a metal spatula, stir-fry until lightly browned but not cooked through, 30 seconds to 1 minute more. Transfer to a plate.

4. Add bok choy and broth to the pan. Cover and cook until the bok choy greens are bright green and almost all the liquid has been absorbed, 1 to 2 minutes. Return the beef to the pan, add the reserved sauce, and stir-fry until the beef is just cooked through and the bok choy is tender-crisp, 30 seconds to 1 minute.

Arugula Salad with Roasted Pork Tenderloin, Pears & Blue Cheese

Ingredients

- 2 tablespoons chopped walnuts

- 3 tablespoons balsamic vinegar

- 2 tablespoons extra-virgin olive oil

- 2 teaspoons lemon juice

- 1 teaspoon honey

- 1 teaspoon Dijon mustard

- 2 teaspoons finely chopped fresh rosemary or 3/4 teaspoon dried

- 1 clove garlic, minced

- ½ teaspoon salt, divided

- ½ teaspoon ground pepper, divided

- 1 pound pork tenderloin

- 8 cups arugula

- 4 small or 2 large red pears, sliced into wedges

- ¼ cup crumbled blue cheese

Directions

1. Preheat oven to 400 degrees F. Coat a large rimmed baking sheet with cooking spray.

2. Cook walnuts in a medium skillet over medium heat, stirring frequently, until golden and fragrant. Set aside.

3. Whisk vinegar, oil, lemon juice, honey, mustard, rosemary, garlic, and 1/4 teaspoon each salt and pepper in a large bowl. Place pork on the prepared baking sheet. Brush with 1 tablespoon

of the dressing and sprinkle with the remaining 1/4 teaspoon each salt and pepper.

4. Roast the pork until a thermometer registers 145 degrees F, 20 to 22 minutes. Transfer to a clean cutting board and let stand for 5 minutes. Cut into slices about 3/4 inch thick.

5. Add arugula and pears to the dressing in the large bowl and toss to coat. Divide the salad among 4 serving plates. Top with pork, cheese, and the reserved walnuts.

Ginger Roasted Salmon & Broccoli

Ingredients

- 1 ½ tablespoons toasted (dark) sesame oil

- 1 ½ tablespoons reduced-sodium tamari

- 1 ½ tablespoons rice vinegar

- 1 tablespoon grated fresh ginger

- ¼ teaspoon salt, divided

- 8 cups large broccoli florets with 2-inch stalks attached (about 1 pound)

- 1 tablespoon molasses

- 1 ¼ pounds wild salmon, cut into 4 portions

- 2 teaspoons toasted sesame seeds

Directions

1. Preheat oven to 425 degrees F. Coat a rimmed baking sheet with cooking spray.

2. Whisk oil, tamari, vinegar, ginger and 1/8 teaspoon salt in a large bowl. Add broccoli and toss to coat. Transfer to the prepared pan using

tongs or a slotted spoon, leaving as much marinade as possible in the bowl. Whisk molasses into the remaining marinade.

3. Roast the broccoli for 5 minutes. Move it to one side of the pan and place salmon on the other side. Season the salmon with the remaining 1/8 teaspoon salt and brush with the molasses glaze. Roast until the salmon is just cooked through, 7 to 10 minutes more. Sprinkle with sesame seeds.

SIDE DISH RECIPES FOR MULTIPLE SCLEROSIS

Cheesy roasted courgettes

Ingredients

• 4 courgettes, halved lengthways

• 250g tub ricotta

• zest 1 lemon

• 1 chilli, deseeded and finely chopped

• handful chopped herbs, such as mint, parsley and basil

• 4 tbsp dried breadcrumbs

Directions

- STEP 1

Heat oven to 200C/180C fan/gas 6. Use a teaspoon to scoop the seeds from the middle of each courgette half, then place them in a large baking tray.

- STEP 2

Mix together the ricotta, zest, chilli and herbs, and season with salt and pepper. Pile the stuffing into the courgettes and top with breadcrumbs. Bake for 35 mins until the courgettes are tender and the topping is golden and crisp.

Baked feta with sesame & honey

Ingredients

- 1 tbsp sesame seeds, toasted

- 200g block feta

- 2 tbsp honey, plus extra to serve

- 1 tsp roughly chopped oregano

- olive oil, for drizzling

- warmed pitta breads, to serve

Directions

- STEP 1

Heat the oven to 200C/180C fan/gas 6, or if using an air-fryer, heat to 180C for 3 mins. Put the sesame seeds in a shallow dish and brush the block of feta all over with the honey. Carefully press the honey-coated feta into the sesame seeds, turning so that it's well crusted with seeds.

- STEP 2

Put the feta in a baking dish (it should fit snugly), then sprinkle over the oregano and a pinch of sea salt. Drizzle with some olive oil. Bake in the oven for 15-20 mins, or cook in the air-fryer for 15 mins until the feta is soft, then drizzle with a little extra honey and serve with the pitta breads on the side.

Smoked haddock & cheddar fishcakes with watercress sauce

Ingredients

- 425g floury potatoes, cut into large chunks

- 1 bay leaf

- 6 peppercorns

- small bunch flat-leaf parsley, leaves and stalks separated

- 225g smoked haddock fillets, skin on (we used dyed haddock to give the mash a lovely golden colour)

- 200g unsmoked haddock fillets, skin on

- 75g mature British cheddar, grated

- 4 spring onions, 0.5 very finely sliced, 0.5 roughly chopped

- 50g plain flour

- 2 medium eggs, beaten

- 100g fresh breadcrumbs

- sunflower oil, for frying

- 50g watercress (weighed after discarding the thickest stalks)

- 4 tbsp rapeseed oil

• 2 lemons, 1 juiced, 1 cut into small wedges to serve (optional)

Directions

• STEP 1

Put the potatoes, bay leaf, peppercorns and parsley stalks in a big pan of cold water. Cover with a lid, bring to the boil and cook for 15 mins until tender. Using a slotted spoon, transfer the potatoes to a colander and leave to steam-dry. Turn the heat down, add the fish and poach gently for 5 mins until it flakes easily. Tip the potatoes into a big bowl and put the fish in the colander to drain for a few mins.

• STEP 2

Add the cheese, some pepper and a little salt to the potatoes and mash well. Flake in about half the fish, discarding the skin and bones, and mash in too. Flake in the remaining fish in big chunks, scatter over the sliced spring onions and gently mix together. Roll the mixture into golf-ball-sized cakes.

• STEP 3

Tip the flour onto a plate and season. Tip the egg and breadcrumbs into 2 shallow bowls each. Roll each fishcake first in the flour, then the egg, then the breadcrumbs. Sit on some parchment-lined trays that fit in your fridge. Chill for at least 1 hr or up to 24 hrs.

• STEP 4

Fill a deep frying pan with 1-2cm of sunflower oil, heat until shimmering, then brown a few fishcakes at a time, turning regularly. If the oil gets too crumby, change halfway through. You can serve them straight away, or cool and chill for up to 24 hrs in the fridge, then simply warm for 30 mins in an oven at 180C/160C fan/ gas 4 before the party.

• STEP 5

Make the dipping sauce up to 1 hr before serving – put the roughly chopped spring onions, the parsley leaves, watercress, rapeseed oil, 2 tbsp lemon juice and 5 tbsp water in a food processor or blender. Whizz to the consistency of single cream.

• STEP 6

Pile the warm fishcakes onto a platter with a bowl of watercress sauce on the side and some lemon wedges for squeezing over, if you like.

Lemon & coriander couscous

Ingredients

- 250g couscous

- grated zest of a lemon

- 2 x 20g packs fresh coriander

- 4 tbsp raisins

- 4 tbsp toasted pine nuts

Directions

- STEP 1

Prepare 250g couscous with boiling water or stock, according to the packet's instructions.

- STEP 2

Add the lemon zest, fresh coriander, raisins and pine nuts. Season well and drizzle with plenty of olive oil. Goes really well with fish or lamb.

Perfect roast potatoes

Ingredients

- 16 potatoes the best ones to use are Desirée, as they hold their shape, but King Edward and Maris Piper are also good

- 2 tbsp plain flour

- 140g goose fat or duck fat or dripping

- 3 tbsp sunflower oil or vegetable oil

Directions

- STEP 1

Heat oven to 190C/fan 170C/gas 5. Peel the potatoes and cut in half; if very large, cut into quarters, or leave whole if they are small. Tip into a saucepan, cover with cold water, then bring to the boil. Set the timer and boil for exactly 2 mins. Drain the potatoes well, then toss in the colander to fluff up their surfaces, sprinkling over the flour as you go.

• STEP 2

Place a large, sturdy roasting tray over a fairly high heat, then tip in the fat and oil. When sizzling, lower in the potatoes carefully, then gently brown in the hot fat for about 5 mins so all the sides are covered with oil.

• STEP 3

Roast undisturbed for 20 mins, then remove from the oven and gently turn them over with a fish slice. Place the tray on the hob to heat the oil, then return to the oven and cook for another 20 mins. Turn again, putting the tray back on the hob to heat the oil. Give them a final 20 mins in the oven, by which time you should have perfect roast potatoes.

Courgette & anchovy salad

Ingredients

- ¼ tsp fennel seed

- juice and zest ½ lemon

- 1 tbsp extra-virgin olive oil, plus extra for drizzling

- 1 garlic clove, crushed

- 1 large courgette, thinly sliced on the diagonal

- 50g rocket

- 2 anchovy fillets, halved

Directions

- STEP 1

Toast the fennel seeds in a small frying pan over a low-medium heat for 1 min, or until they release their aroma. Bash them lightly using a pestle and mortar. Mix the lemon juice, fennel seeds, oil and garlic in a large bowl, then stir in the courgette. Season and set aside to marinate for 30 mins.

- STEP 2

Toss through the rocket and transfer to a platter. Top with the anchovy fillets. Scatter with lemon zest and serve with an extra drizzle of olive oil.

Barbecued fennel with black olive dressing

Ingredients

- 2 fennel bulbs, sliced lengthways into 1cm-thick pieces

- 1 ½ tbsp olive oil

- 2 tbsp finely chopped black Kalamata olive

- 1 garlic clove, crushed

- juice 1 lemon

- small handful each parsley and basil, finely chopped

Directions

- STEP 1

Heat a BBQ or griddle pan. Toss the fennel in 1 tbsp of the oil, coating well. Cook for 5 mins on each side until golden brown and charred.

• STEP 2

To make the dressing, put the olives, garlic, lemon juice and remaining oil in a bowl. Add the chopped herbs and combine. Lay the fennel on a platter and pour over the dressing. Eat warm or at room temperature.

Apricot pancakes with honey butter

Ingredients

For the butter

• 100g butter, softened

• 2 tbsp clear honey

For the pancakes

- 140g self-raising flour

- pinch bicarbonate of soda

- 25g caster sugar

- 1 egg

- 150ml milk

- handful ready-to-eat dried apricots, finely chopped

- oil, for frying

Directions

- STEP 1

For the honey butter, beat the butter with the honey and spoon onto a large piece of cling film.

Squeeze into a sausage shape, then wrap tightly and chill until ready to use. Will keep in the fridge for up to a month.

• STEP 2

Sift the flour, bicarbonate of soda and a small pinch of salt into a bowl, then stir through the sugar and make a well in the centre. Beat together the egg and milk, then gradually pour into the well, stirring slowly, to avoid creating lumps. Stir in the apricots.

• STEP 3

Heat a non-stick frying pan over a low heat and add a little oil. Drop in 4 tablespoonfuls of batter and cook for 1 min or until the surface of each pancake is covered in bubbles. Flip with a palette knife or fish slice, then cook for a further min. Repeat with the remaining batter. Serve warm or leave to cool, then toast and spread with the honey butter to serve

Harissa cauliflower pilaf

Ingredients

- 300g basmati rice

- 1 red onion, finely sliced

- 2 lemons, 1 juiced, 1 cut into wedges

- 2 tsp sugar

- 4 tbsp harissa

- 1 garlic clove, crushed

- 1 tbsp olive oil

- 1 large or 2 medium cauliflower, broken into large florets, stalk chopped, large leaves roughly chopped

- pinch of saffron

- 2 bay leaves

- 700ml hot vegan vegetable stock

- 100g sultanas

- 100g flaked almonds, toasted until golden brown

- ½ small bunch of dill, chopped, plus extra to serve

- 400g can chickpeas, drained and rinsed

- 50g pomegranate seeds (optional)

Directions

- STEP 1

Wash the rice really well, then leave to soak in cold water for 1 hr. Put the onion in a small bowl and toss with the lemon juice, the sugar and a pinch of salt. Leave to pickle while you make the pilaf.

- STEP 2

Heat the oven to 200C/180C fan/gas 6. Whisk 2 tbsp harissa, the garlic and oil in a large bowl, then add the cauliflower and toss to coat in the sauce. Season, then tip into a roasting tin and roast for 30 mins until tender and golden.

- STEP 3

Meanwhile, mix the saffron, bay leaves, stock and 2 tbsp harissa in a pan over a very low heat to keep warm while the cauli roasts.

- STEP 4

Remove the cauli from the oven, tip into a dish and squeeze over the juice from one of the lemon wedges. Drain the rice and tip into the roasting tin. Pour over the infused stock, and mix well. Stir in the sultanas, half the almonds, the dill, chickpeas, and half the cauliflower. Cover the tin with a double layer of foil, sealing well, then bake for 30 mins until the rice is tender and stock is absorbed.

- STEP 5

Fluff up the rice with a fork, then fold in the remaining cauliflower (this creates a contrast of cauli textures). Scatter over the extra dill, the remaining almonds, the pomegranate seeds, if using, the pickled red onions and remaining lemon wedges to squeeze over.

Quinoa, pea & avocado salad

Ingredients

- 100g frozen peas

- juice 1 lemon

- 2 tbsp olive oil

- ½ small pack mint, leaves only, chopped

- ½ small pack chives, snipped

- 250g pack ready-to-eat red & white quinoa mix (we used Merchant Gourmet)

- 1 avocado, stoned, peeled and chopped into chunks

- 75g bag pea shoots

Directions

• STEP 1

Put the peas in a large heatproof bowl, pour over just-boiled water, then set aside.

• STEP 2

Pour the lemon juice into a small bowl and whisk in some seasoning. Keep whisking as you slowly add the olive oil, followed by the mint and chives.

• STEP 3

Drain the peas and tip into a large serving dish. Stir in the quinoa, breaking up any clumps. Pour over the dressing, then fold in the avocado and pea shoots. Serve immediately.

Spicy salmon tabbouleh

Ingredients

- 400g bulgur wheat

- 500g salmon fillet, pin-boned

- 3 tbsp sunflower oil

- 2 onions, finely chopped

- 5cm piece ginger, peeled and finely chopped

- 2 tbsp curry paste (we used korma)

- 300g Greek yogurt

- juice 1 lemon, plus 2 cut into wedges, to serve

- 300g smoked salmon

- handful coriander or parsley, roughly chopped

Directions

- STEP 1

Cook the bulgur wheat in plenty of salted water for 7 mins (or follow pack instructions). Drain, tip into a large bowl and leave to cool. Put the salmon fillet on a foil-lined grill, brush lightly with oil and season. Grill for 7-10 mins, turning halfway, until the fish flakes easily. Cool.

• STEP 2

Heat the remaining oil, add the onions and ginger, and fry for about 5 mins until softened and lightly coloured. Stir in the curry paste and cook for 1 min, stirring. Remove from the heat and stir in the yogurt, lemon juice and some seasoning. Leave to cool.

• STEP 3

Skin and flake the salmon fillet. Cut the smoked salmon into strips. Add the fresh salmon and half the smoked salmon to the bulgur wheat with the dressing and half the coriander. Stir everything together lightly, so as not to break up the salmon flakes too much. Tip onto a serving platter and scatter over the remaining smoked salmon strips and coriander. Add the lemon wedges and serve.

Warm mackerel & beetroot salad

Ingredients

- 450g new potato, cut into bite-size pieces

- 3 smoked mackerel fillets, skinned

- 250g pack cooked beetroot

- 100g bag mixed salad leaves

- 2 celery sticks, finely sliced

- 50g walnut pieces

For the dressing

- 6 tbsp good-quality salad dressing

- 2 tsp creamed horseradish sauce

Directions

- STEP 1

Boil the potatoes for 12-15 mins until just tender. Meanwhile, flake the mackerel fillets into large pieces and cut the beetroot into bite-size chunks.

- STEP 2

Drain the potatoes and cool slightly. Mix the salad dressing and horseradish sauce together in a salad bowl and season. Tip in the potatoes – they should still be warm.

- STEP 3

Add the salad leaves, mackerel, beetroot, celery and walnuts, and toss gently. Serve with crusty bread.

Courgettes with mint & ricotta

Ingredients

- 2 tbsp olive oil

- 2 tsp unsalted butter

- 4 large courgettes (we used a mixture of green and yellow), sliced

- zest and juice 1 lemon

- pinch of chilli flakes

- 70g ricotta

- extra virgin olive oil, for drizzling

• handful mint leaves, picked and roughly chopped

Directions

• STEP 1

Heat a large, heavy non-stick frying pan or cast-iron skillet over a medium heat. Heat 1 tbsp of the oil and 1 tsp butter together and add half the courgettes in one layer. Cook for 2 mins, then turn the heat down to medium-low and cook for 5 more mins untouched, until the underside has a nice colour. Flip the courgettes, then grate over some lemon zest, pour over half the lemon juice and season with salt, pepper and chilli flakes. Cook for a further 5 mins or until very tender. Repeat the process with the remaining slices of courgette.

• STEP 2

Transfer to a platter and top with spoonfuls of ricotta. Drizzle over some extra virgin olive oil and scatter over the mint to serve.

Stir-fried greens with fish sauce

Ingredients

- ½ head Savoy cabbage

- 125g purple sprouting or Tenderstem broccoli

- 2 tbsp groundnut oil

- 4-6 garlic cloves, finely sliced

- 75g baby spinach

- 2 tbsp fish sauce, plus extra for seasoning

- 1 tsp caster sugar

Directions

• STEP 1

Remove any discoloured or coarse leaves from the cabbage, then halve it. Remove the hard central ribs and discard them, then shred the leaves. If using purple sprouting broccoli, halve any thicker stems lengthways.

• STEP 2

Heat the oil in a wok. Stir-fry the broccoli for 1 min, then add the garlic and cabbage and cook until the garlic is a pale gold colour. Quickly add the spinach and fish sauce and turn the veg over – the moisture should come out of the spinach and boil off quickly. Add the sugar and toss the vegetables again, then add a little more fish sauce, if you like.

Fish o'leekie

Ingredients

* 1 leek, finely sliced

* 500ml vegetable stock

* 300g basmati rice

* 500g cod or haddock fillet, skinned and cut into large chunks

* handful parsley, roughly chopped

* finely grated zest and juice 1 lemon

Directions

* STEP 1

Put the leek in a large microwave dish with 4 tbsp of the stock. Cover the dish with cling film, pierce the film with a knife, then microwave on High for 5 mins.

• STEP 2

Uncover the dish, then stir the rice and remaining stock into the leek. Re-cover with cling film, pierce and microwave on High for another 10 mins, stirring halfway through until the rice is very nearly cooked.

• STEP 3

Gently stir in the fish chunks, cover the dish with cling film again, then pierce and cook for a further 5 mins until the fish flakes easily and the rice is tender. Stir in the parsley, lemon zest and juice. Leave to stand for 2 mins before serving.

PART V

LIVING WITH MS

Tips to Ease MS Symptoms

You can do a few things that may ease multiple sclerosis symptoms:

Prioritize sleep. Make sure you're getting quality sleep and enough of it. Keep consistent sleep and wake times to maintain good sleep hygiene. If you have obstructive sleep apnea or another sleep disorder, talk to your doctor about treating it.

Eat well. Nutrition plays a role in health, so a balanced diet can help you feel your best. Eat whole grains instead of refined grains. Avoid or limit processed foods and added sugar. Eat plenty of fruits and veggies.

Exercise regularly. Getting active regularly may enhance your strength, balance, and coordination.

Keep cool. Symptoms can get worse if your body temperature is higher. Avoid the heat, or wear clothing that helps you stay cool.

Destress. Stress can trigger symptoms, so find a way to relieve stress that works for you. Yoga, meditation, or massage may help.

Avoid smoking. This is linked to a wide range of diseases and conditions. Smoking can also make MS symptoms get worse more quickly.

Get regular care. See your doctor or health care professional regularly to keep tabs on symptoms. Ask for information on new and upcoming treatments.

Customize your environment. Make whatever modifications you need in your living spaces to accommodate your multiple sclerosis. That may mean things including decluttering, adding grab bars, and other adjustments.

Anticipate possible changes. MS may change how much you can work (and it can stop you from being able to work). As a result, you may earn less (or not be able to earn an income at all). In one study, people with MS who had lower socioeconomic status became disabled faster. Participants were more likely to experience SPMS which means their neurologic function got worse more quickly, too.

Seek support. Connecting with others who have MS may give you the mental and emotional support needed to live well.

Lifestyle and Home Remedies

To help relieve the signs and symptoms of MS, try to:

Get plenty of rest. Look at your sleep habits to make sure you're getting the best possible sleep. To make sure you're getting enough sleep, you may need to be evaluated — and possibly treated — for sleep disorders such as obstructive sleep apnea.

Exercise. If you have mild to moderate MS, regular exercise can help improve your strength, muscle tone, balance and coordination. Swimming or other water exercises are good options if you have intolerance to heat. Other types of mild to moderate exercise recommended for people with MS include walking, stretching, low-impact aerobics, stationary bicycling, yoga and tai chi.

Cool down. MS symptoms may worsen when the body temperature rises in some people with MS. Avoiding exposure to heat and using devices such as cooling scarves or vests can be helpful.

Eat a balanced diet. Since there is little evidence to support a particular diet, experts recommend a generally healthy diet. Some research suggests that vitamin D may have potential benefit for people with MS.

Relieve stress. Stress may trigger or worsen your signs and symptoms. Yoga, tai chi, massage, meditation or deep breathing may help.

Alternative Medicine

Many people with MS use a variety of alternative or complementary treatments or both to help manage their symptoms, such as fatigue and muscle pain.

Activities such as exercise, meditation, yoga, massage, eating a healthier diet, acupuncture and relaxation techniques may help boost overall mental and physical well-being in patients with MS.

According to guidelines from the American Academy of Neurology, research strongly indicates that oral cannabis extract (OCE) may improve symptoms of muscle spasticity and pain. There is a lack of evidence that cannabis in any other form is effective in managing other MS symptoms.

Daily intake of vitamin D3 of 2,000 to 5,000 international units daily is recommended in those with MS. The connection between vitamin D and MS is supported by the association with exposure to sunlight and the risk of MS.

Coping and Support

Living with any chronic illness can be difficult. To manage the stress of living with MS, consider these suggestions:

Maintain normal daily activities as best you can.

Stay connected to friends and family.

Continue to pursue hobbies that you enjoy and are able to do.

Contact a support group, for yourself or for family members.

Discuss your feelings and concerns about living with MS with your doctor or a counselor.